STILLBIRTH AND MISCARRIAGE, A LIFE-CHANGING LOSS

'Say my baby's name'

T0054416

An important book for anyone involved in maternity care. Death in the context of pregnancy, and the surrounding depths of human emotions, have a direct and clear patient voice here. This is a re-education on the exquisite importance of human kindness in the clinical setting.

Cathy Allen, Consultant Obstetrician Gynaecologist in charge of the Recurrent Pregnancy Loss Clinic, National Maternity Hospital, Dublin

This book gives voice to the cry from the heart of mothers, fathers and siblings bereaved by the loss of a baby. It challenges our long-standing societal taboos and the tragic legacy of the *cillíní* (historic burial sites in Ireland, primarily used for stillborn and unbaptised infants). It is essential reading for professionals involved in the care of our babies, their parents and their families.

Máirín O'Donovan, Principal Social Worker and Family Therapist working with HSE West Cork Child and Adolescent Mental Health

The great thing about this book is that it values listening to parents who have lost or are losing a child to miscarriage or stillbirth, hearing their pain and responding to their actual needs rather than the hospital's idea of what their needs should be.

It ought to be prescribed reading for all health professionals who have anything to do with looking after women during pregnancy and when they are giving birth.

It is full of heartbreak, bewilderment, anger, but also love, gratitude and even joy. It is also full of practical suggestions about how a devastating experience can be handled with empathy, kindness and support – which can make the difference between an experience that is deeply sad and one that is utterly traumatising.

Siobhán Parkinson, former Children's Laureate and author of *All Shining in the Spring* (a stillbirth story for children, recently reissued by Little Island Books)

Working in women's health has brought me into contact with couples who have suffered the loss of a baby, one of the most challenging aspects of our work. Dr Anne Tracey's book offers us a deep and privileged insight into what women, men and families experience at all stages of pregnancy when a baby dies, and those affected by such a profound loss. It is a credit to those who have shared their lived experiences for the benefit of others. The simple act of speaking their child's name can be a powerful acknowledgement. I wholeheartedly recommend this book to both professionals and general readers.

Kevin Glackin, Consultant Obstetrician and Gynaecologist at Western Health and Social Care Trust with special interest in high-risk pregnancy and fetal medicine

The emotional impact that pregnancy loss and stillbirth can have on parents is vividly presented in Anne Tracey's book. Based on interviews with five men and twenty-seven women, Dr Tracey elicits what the journey from conception to loss can entail. Many people who have experienced pregnancy loss or stillbirth, as well as their family and friends, will find this book helpful and informative.

Rosanne Cecil, Editor of *The Anthropology of Pregnancy Loss: Comparative studies in miscarriage, stillbirth and neonatal death*

Thank you for giving voice to the parents who spoke so openly and honestly about their loss. It is a beautiful and fitting acknowledgement of the pain and grief experienced by many people living among us who have lost a baby through stillbirth or miscarriage. The recommendations at the end of the book, rooted in the preceding narratives and personal stories of the men and women involved, provide much food for thought and even more for action. The book brings hope to readers and highlights the way in which honouring their baby, in whatever way was right for them, brought some comfort and consolation to the parents in this book.

Professor Assumpta Ryan, Ulster University

Titles in the *MindYourSelf* Mental Health and Well-Being Series

STILLBIRTH AND MISCARRIAGE, A LIFE-CHANGING LOSS

'Say my baby's name'

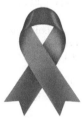

Dr Anne Tracey
SERIES EDITOR: Dr Marie Murray

ATRIUM

First published in 2022 by Atrium
Atrium is an imprint of Cork University Press
Boole Library
University College Cork
Cork T12 ND89
Ireland

Library of Congress Control Number: 2022942672

Distribution in the USA Longleaf Services, Chapel Hill,
NC, USA.

British Library Cataloguing in Publication Data
A CIP catalogue record for this book is available from the
British Library.

ISBN 9781782055273

Design and typesetting by Studio 10 Design
Printed by HussarBooks in Poland

www.corkuniversitypress.com

DR MARIE MURRAY has worked as a clinical psychologist for more than forty years across the entire developmental spectrum. An honours graduate of UCD, from where she also obtained an MSc and PhD, she is a chartered psychologist, registered family therapist and supervisor, a member of both the Irish Council for Psychotherapy and the European Association for Psychotherapy, as well as the APA American Psychological Association and a former member of the Heads of Psychology Services in Ireland. Key clinical posts have included being Director of Psychology in St Vincent's Psychiatric Hospital Dublin and Director of Student Counselling Services in UCD. Marie served on the Medical Council of Ireland (2008–13) and on the Council of the Psychological Society of Ireland (2014–17) She has presented internationally, from the Tavistock and Portman NHS Trust in London to (PKU) Peking University, Beijing. She was an *Irish Times* columnist for eight years and has been author, co-author, contributor and editor to a number of bestselling books, many with accompanying RTÉ radio programmes. Her appointment as Series Editor to Cork University Press *MindYourSelf* series gathers a lifetime of professional experience to bring safe clinical information to general and professional readers.

Stillbirth and Miscarriage, a Life-changing Loss: 'Say my baby's name' is dedicated to all of you who have experienced the loss of a precious baby. Here we remember every little lost life that had their existence and were present for a short time on this earth. Each of you remain in our hearts, forever.

In memory of my beloved parents, Francis and Susan Corey, Moneymore, County Derry.

CONTENTS

DISCLAIMER

This book has been written for general readers to introduce the topic or to increase their knowledge and understanding of it. It is not intended, or implied, to be a substitute for professional consultation or advice in this, or allied areas. Any content, text, graphics, images or other information provided in any of the *MindYourSelf* books is for general purposes only.

On topics that have medical, psychological, psychiatric, psycho-therapy, nursing, physiotherapy, occupational therapy, educational, vocational, organisational, sociological, legal or any mental health- or physical health-related or other content, *MindYourSelf* books do not replace diagnosis, treatment or any other appropriate professional consultations and interventions. This also applies to any informa-tion or website links contained in the book.

While every effort has been made to ensure the accuracy of the information in the book, it is possible that errors or omissions may occur. Research also leads to new multidisciplinary perspectives in all professional areas, so that despite all the publishers' caution and care, new thinking on certain topics may alter the accuracy of the content. The authors, editors and publishers can, therefore, assume no responsibility, nor provide any guarantees or warranties concern-ing the up-to-date nature of the information provided.

The views expressed in the book are solely those of the author and of the participants in the research. To preserve the anonymity of the research participants, their names have been changed. The names of living children have been omitted and other identifying details have been excluded. However, the testimony of the participants told directly from their hearts is preserved – their words, their stories, their feelings and emotions, which they have so generously shared and which it is hoped will serve to enlighten, guide and comfort readers.

MindYourSelf

Few expressions convey as much care as that lovely phrase 'mind yourself'. Quintessentially Irish, it is a blessing, an injunction, an endearment and a solicitous farewell. Like many simple phrases, 'mind yourself' has layers of psychological meaning, so that while it trips lightly off the tongue at the end of conversations, there are depths of kindness that accompany it.

Being told to 'mind yourself' touches the heart. It resonates with the longing in each of us to have somebody in our world who cares about us. Saying 'mind yourself' means 'you matter to me'; that what happens to you is important, and may nothing bad befall you. It is a cautionary phrase, with a gentle acknowledgement of your personal responsibility in self-care. Although it has become so ingrained in our leave-taking that we may not consciously note it, unconsciously, being minded is an atavistic need in all of us. 'Mind yourself' is what parents say to children, to adolescents, what people say to each other, to family and friends. We also say it to reassure ourselves that we have reminded those we love to keep themselves safe.

It is in this spirit of recognising the importance of self-care that the *MindYourSelf* book series has been designed; to bring safe, researched, peer-reviewed information from front-line professionals to help people to mind themselves. While, at one level, information – about everything – is now on multiple platforms at the touch of a screen, relying on internet sites is a problem. What is true? Who can you trust? How do you sift through the data to find what you need to know? Because it is not lack of access to facts, but fact overload, that makes people increasingly conscious of the dangers of misinformation, contradictory perspectives, internet prognoses and the risk of unreliable or exploitative sources. What people want is simply the information that is relevant to them, delivered by professionals who care about their specialities and who are keen to help readers understand the topic. May this Cork University Press *MindYourSelf* series find its way to all who need it, and give readers the tools and resources to really mind themselves.

Dr Marie Murray, Series Editor, *MindYourSelf*

NOTES ON PARTICIPANTS

Áine

I am a university lecturer and academic married to a wonderful man. Following the loss of our baby, we have been blessed with two healthy children. I truly hope that in sharing my experience in this book, others will be helped.

Amy

I am a busy mother working in the field of education. I took part in the study to give people insight into the experience of life during recurrent miscarriage; how all-encompassing it can be and how miscarriage impacts on every member of the family. My message to readers is one of hope, that they will find solace in this book and that it is a reminder to women who have had a miscarriage that they are not alone.

Anna

I'm Anna. We are a family living on the north coast of Northern Ireland but one of our children, Gerry, 'got away'; baby Gerry was born at thirty-two weeks. Our children are a wonderful bunch but there is always one missing and there is a special place in our hearts for the beautiful boy we lost. We want him to be remembered, he is so much a part of our family.

Bernadette

Married to my soulmate and with our beautiful children, we have also had the privilege of being parents to five other little heartbeats that unfortunately we did not get to meet but they are very much part of our beautiful family. I was so pleased to participate in Anne's study as I believe that miscarriage is still considered a taboo subject and so families grieve in silence. Bereaved families should be allowed to honour their little ones, no matter how long or short a time they were with them. I hope that readers who have not experienced this type of loss will get an insight into the heartbreak, loneliness and emptiness that is caused by a miscarriage. For readers who have tragically suffered a miscarriage, I hope it will comfort you to know that your grief is normal and you are not alone. Thanks to Anne for allowing us all to tell our stories and for shining a light on a very difficult issue.

Beth

I am a mother, writer and academic born in the beautiful state of Maine, USA, and studied in Washington, DC. When my husband and I moved to Ireland it was supposedly for one year, but we never left! I come from a long line of women who have lost pregnancies and infants, and I am grateful to have been part of a book which gives a space to express grief and to invite other families to feel less alone.

Bridget

Our journey to parenthood was horrendous: long, emotional and mostly sad. I never felt emotional pain like it in my life. Losing fifteen babies as we did has torn an irreplaceable part of my heart away. Unless you have been on a similar journey you could never imagine the pain. It took thirteen long, hard years but we got there and we have two beautiful children. My advice is: listen to your heart. I knew that one day I would have my own child, I just had to get over all the hurdles day by day and year on year. Never say never. Good luck to all those on their journey, stay strong.

Cecilia

I am the mother of four beautiful children and a beautiful angel baby girl, Alex. There is a taboo around losing a child and people often don't know how to act or talk to you so they avoid you instead. Since Alex's passing life has been tough, each day is an uphill battle, which I think may continue for the rest of my life. When we celebrate a milestone, birthday or event I think of how much we have missed and dreamed for our lost child. If taking part in this research and talking about my loss helps one person or helps change the response to this very sensitive topic, my pain will not have been in vain.

Drew

Following a miscarriage and a stillbirth my wife and I went on to have two healthy children. We do everything we can to improve support for bereaved parents and help to reduce stillbirth rates. I am passionate about increasing the voices of fathers in conversations around child bereavement. I am pleased to be a part of this publication which provides an authentic platform for parents to share their experience and hope it will lead to an increase in confidence for those supporting people affected by the loss of a child.

Eimear

I am the proud mother of two grown-up children. For twenty years I have provided vocational guidance to people. Taking part in this book provided the opportunity for me to talk about my third child, whom I've never met. The experiences shared in this book highlight the emotional impact of the loss of a baby.

Gabrielle

I am married with one son. Being active, fit and healthy, I never envisaged any trouble having a baby. I was pregnant five times and feel the 'weight' of the loss of each unborn child. I hope by giving voice to the pain of loss that it will be helpful to those working in the medical arena and to people who want to know more about the emotional and physical impact of miscarriage and stillbirth.

Grace

A researcher and health professional, I am also a mum and a step-mum. I have a cascade of stars tattooed on my body representing the people who have lit my way, including my husband and his children, and I have two smaller stars which represent my children, Caoimhe and Daniel, who did not get to be born. My babies have left their footprints forever on my heart and will never be forgotten as long as I live.

Jane

I am an artist and married with three children. Before having my children I suffered a miscarriage and always felt that there was a lack of support for women in these circumstances, especially the 'silence' that often surrounds baby loss. I wanted my story to help others. What I didn't anticipate was the cathartic benefits that taking part in the book would have, the emotions that came to the surface that surprised me and helped me to 'let go' of a lot relating to the miscarriage. I hope that this book will help medical practitioners to improve the treatment of women in hospital. You never forget the people who are kind and compassionate. Doctors and nurses have 'seen it all before' but women are devastated by loss.

John and Emily

Married for two decades, we have three children but sadly our daughter Caoimhe was stillborn. We wanted to share our story of loss in the hope that other parents, who may have gone through the same difficult journey, would feel that they are not alone. Supporting our other children in age-appropriate ways, we included them particularly when their sister Caoimhe came home so that they understood what was happening. Also becoming involved in Féileacáin has given us the platform through which we can honour the memory of Caoimhe by reaching out to others in need of help.

Kathy (Tribute to Kathy RIP by her husband Ernest)

To me, there was no-one quite like Kathy; she was truly one of a kind. We were made for each other. God's love shone from her wherever she went with her infectious beaming smile. She always had a listening ear and she thought more of others than herself despite her own health problems. She truly had the spirit of God within her. Now she is in the presence of the Lord rejoicing with the children she lost, and her family and friends who departed before her. I will never forget my soul mate who lives on in my heart, in my memories, and in the wonderful legacy of our miracle child

Leo and Gretta

We were a professional couple with two young children when we experienced the devastating loss of our twins. There will always be that void in our family but it has made us truly thankful for the children that we did get to rear. The first time as a couple that we discussed this was on our way to do the interviews for the book, almost ten years after it had happened. The pain is still raw and every detail as clear as it was when it happened. I think you just get better at keeping the lid on it. It catches you some days when you least expect it and all you can do is wait for it to pass. This book is an important one that should be widely read. It powerfully illustrates the experiential variation miscarriage is, and the hauntingly personal toll it takes on each individual.

Lilly

My daughter Amilia Rose was stillborn. Two years later my son was born; a saviour. He enriched my life with love, hope and fulfilment. This book expresses the pain we have all gone through. People need to understand the severity of having a baby die. If you are reading this book following a stillbirth or miscarriage, I hope you know you are not alone and that your baby will never be forgotten. I would like to take this opportunity to thank Dr Tracey for her commitment and compassion in researching such a sensitive and important subject.

Maria

I am married to Archie and I am the mother of three children. Our baby Sam was delivered at twenty-four weeks, an experience that was distressing and painful. We have found beautiful ways to remember and honour our child which you will read about in the book. I hope by telling our story that you, the reader, will find solace and comfort in knowing that you are not alone.

Mary

I have been married to Liam for twenty years and we have three children who are a joy to us. Our son Emmet Pio was delivered at twenty-five weeks and did not survive. We remember him every day and will miss him forever. When I read through the chapters of this book, I was honoured to see the stories – sad and painful as they are – in print for others to read. It is a truly informative read for those who wish to learn more about the short- and long-term impact of stillbirth and miscarriage on a family.

Maura

My children brought me great consolation in the difficult times after losing Ronan. I can resonate with the stories of other mums and dads who have experienced the heartbreak of loss. I want the readers of this book to know that the days, weeks and months after losing a baby are dark. As time goes on, normality begins to filter back. They say time is a healer and things do get easier but there's always the wonder of what our life would be like if Ronan was here; if all our little angels were able to stay with us.

Rose

My job is in an academic setting. I am married to Gerard and we have four children: Ellen, who was stillborn at thirty-nine weeks, her two brothers and her sister. The key message I would like to convey to anyone expecting a child or thinking of starting a family is this: 'Listen to your instincts and make sure that your instincts are listened to.'

Ruth

Hello reader. I am mum to six children with my husband. Five of our children are living and well but I lost one of our babies nine weeks into my pregnancy. It was a shocking and distressing experience, especially the way it all happened, which you will read about in the chapters of this book. I wanted to tell my story so that lessons could be learned from what we went through and that in some way it would be a support to other bereaved parents out there.

Sarrah

I am the mother of six children: Grace the little baby I lost and five grown-up children. I am also grandmother to gorgeous grandbabies, the eldest of whom was born days after I lost Grace. I choose to celebrate and be thankful for Grace's life every day because, even though she is no longer physically with me, she is in my heart every second of every day.

Serena

I am a mum who works in education. My miscarriage was labelled a mis-miscarriage, which was something I had never heard of until the day of my first scan at fourteen weeks. Apparently, the baby had died a few weeks before my scan but my body had not registered this. I made the decision to bring the remains home and bury my baby; it was a comfort to have a place to visit. My children all know about their sibling. I found that if I spoke about the miscarriage, some people said nothing, while for others who opened up talking was a release as they had told no one else outside of their family.

Shauna

Married with four children, our second daughter Branna was stillborn and is our angel in heaven. She weighed 8 lb 6 oz and looked perfect in every way. I hope parents will take some comfort from reading about our experiences and know that they are not alone. Every single feeling experienced throughout this traumatic time is completely normal. We never forget, yet time is a healer and things do get easier. It is good to talk about your baby and share your experience with others. Our baby is part of our family and we keep her memory alive. Much love to all who are reading this book – you are all in my thoughts.

Tara

I am a lecturer at a local university and happily married. I have a young son who was born after the two miscarriages that are discussed in this book. I truly hope that others will find comfort and solace in the experiences shared here.

Tess

Growing up, I thought of becoming a mammy as an integral part of life. I count myself very lucky to have three little angels awaiting me and two beautiful earth children. My losses have taught me so much about who the true stars in life are: my husband, a rock despite his own grief journey, and my family and friends. During my struggles, the support of my big sister (who understood the pain of miscarriage) and of my husband are the reasons I am still here. Sadly, since participating in this book, my sister has died. I love and miss my beautiful sister, every day.

Tony and Betty

We have three children: Joshua, who was stillborn, and two rainbow babies ('rainbow' babies are 'babies that follow loss'). It was a complete shock when we were told that Joshua's heart had stopped beating. His birth was silent; we knew we would never hear him cry. No parent ever expects this, so the rainbow pregnancies were full of anxiety. Having another baby does not 'fix' things because despite the love our living children bring to our lives, there is a hole that cannot be filled and Joshua will always be a part of our family. Supporting other parents has helped us. Baby loss should not be a taboo subject. The most important thing that people can do is remember children who have died: just say their name.

Willie and Catherine

We were happily married for a year when we found out we were expecting a baby. That pregnancy went well, and we assumed that the next pregnancy would be just as smooth. Little did we know that the rollercoaster ride, that you will read about in this book, was just beginning. We believe in hope and in persevering. We hope this book will help and support you.

FOREWORD

The death of a baby is an acute, excruciating loss experienced at the most profound level of being. Regardless of what stage in pregnancy the loss occurs, the trauma for parents is deep; a depth excavated exquisitely by Dr Anne Tracey, psychologist, researcher and author of this beautiful book *Stillbirth and Miscarriage, a Life-changing Loss: 'Say my baby's name'*.

The book is based on Dr Tracey's all-Ireland study via in-depth interviews with parents who have suffered life-changing loss through stillbirth and miscarriage. It is *their* stories, *their* voices that we hear. From the first happy moments when pregnancy is confirmed, to feelings of foreboding that something may be wrong, on to the devastating loss at different stages of the pregnancy, the stories unfold and with them our understanding and insight into life-changing loss.

When I first read the text I was impressed by the depth and wealth of information the book contained. But more than that, I was moved by the stories. As I came to know the narrators, to hear their voices, to understand their pain and to appreciate the individuality of their accounts, my admiration grew. Many had suffered multiple losses. Others had a single account. Some already had children; others went on to have rainbow babies, though sadly for some that did not occur. But all of them describe being traumatised in one way or another; all had suffered extremely and yet found it in their grieving hearts to share their stories for the benefit of others. And so I formed a connection with them and with their babies whom I will hold in my own heart forever.

Stillbirth and Miscarriage, a Life-changing Loss: 'Say my baby's name' begins with Dr Tracey's own awareness of her parents 'drenched' in sorrow at the loss of their beautiful son Patrick; an experience which no doubt was to influence Dr Tracey's own distinguished career path. Therefore this book is not just based on the rigour of an experienced researcher, the insights of a fine psychologist, or the work of an accomplished author but the empathy of a practitioner who knows about loss first hand and who brings us the accounts of the interviewees who trust her as they share their stories stoically and generously with her, and through her with all of us.

One of the distinguishing features of the book is that the chapter titles are based on direct quotes from the parents as their stories unfold. Most of the accounts are so raw and real that they are difficult to read but they bring us into the lived reality of stillbirth and miscarriage from which we gain insights essential for anyone who wishes to understand. In so doing, the parents gift their knowledge and expertise to readers and to multidisciplinary professionals who may not know the secret wounds of previous loss carried by people they meet.

The chapter titles guide us through the book.

- From Chapter 1 we understand that *As soon as you know you are pregnant, the relationship begins.*

- Chapter 2 introduces the realisation that all may not be well, that *Something was wrong.*

- The dreaded confirmation arises in Chapter 3, *I am sorry, I cannot get a heartbeat.*

- In Chapter 4 we encounter the all-consuming longing to hold a baby in *My body was screaming 'baby'* – a harrowing and heartbreaking read.

- There is the primeval terror of Chapter 5's question, *Why did my baby die?*, to which no human answer is adequate.

- In Chapter 6, *The silence was deafening*, we feel the clinical chill when a baby is born without life, the deadly silence of the stillborn. It is a cruel paradox, the absence of presence, that the stillborn is lost to the mother at the moment of birth.

In the words of Seamus Heaney, this is the 'evicted world' when the baby is expelled from life and the mother is left steeped in grief at the empty chasm of her womb.

But the book does not dwell exclusively on mothers, nor does it forget the fathers who stand in delivery rooms watching their wives or partners in distress. Men, too often presumed to be invulnerable to the intensity of what is happening, find even fewer places in which their stories of disappointment, fear, anger, grief and longing can be heard. Fortunately in Chapter 10, titled *Men are not in the line of vision*, their accounts are heard, and importantly the book also addresses the impact on siblings and the entire extended family in practical ways.

Because the emotions that accompany grief are complex, when babies die before they are born complexity is increased. It must be therapeutic that the book describes anger, and envy towards others who are pregnant: … *it was awful. I hated her so much. All my family were congratulating her … I was jealous of her. It's okay to feel that way.*

The wheels of guilt are also unrelenting, with the inevitable question, *Why could my body not carry my baby, what did I do wrong?* Guilt is heightened because many mothers speak about a deep visceral knowing when the life of their baby begins; the attachment that occurs from the moment they know they are pregnant; the love for a little life struggling to survive; the sound on a sonogram, the acute sense of failure when their bodies betray them, so that they could not hold on to and protect the potentiality of that life.

It is no surprise then, that miscarriage and stillbirth can be the 'loneliest' experiences in the world; or how anxious, ill, angry and depressed, traumatised parents may become. Parents may grieve differently which can drive them apart. Children can find their lives eclipsed if their parents descend into grief or become hypervigilant and overprotective of them.

But we also learn from the book that there are 'saviours' out there, individuals, support systems and organisations (see the 'Other Resources' section in the book) to help parents cope; how beautifully children try to console their parents; how united some families can become and the extraordinary ways in which parents include the 'imaginary being', their lost baby's meticulous perfection, the life that should have been memorialised in their own lives forever.

Stillbirth and Miscarriage, a Life-changing Loss: 'Say my baby's name' is a work of astonishing pathos, grace, practicality and purpose, containing invaluable information for general readers and professionals on life-changing loss. It is a comprehensive guide through the physical, psychological, emotional, spiritual and practical issues that arise. It reminds readers that these little souls are integral to the life of their parents; that for parents the loss of a pregnancy is the loss of their hopes, their dreams and the future they imagined, now changed utterly and forever. As the title of this book conveys, parents do not want people to shy away from talking about miscarriage and stillbirth but to 'say' their baby's name. They want their child to be recognised, to be spoken about, to live in memory forever.

This book is more than an informative text. It is a tribute to all those who died before birth, to their parents who yearned for them; who did what they could to keep them and who continue to honour, commemorate and remember them. The length of a life may be but a positive line on a pregnancy test, a fluttering in the womb, a moment, a heartbeat or a single breath, but it matters to those who loved them and the people they might have become.

It has been my privilege to edit this book and to write this Foreword. Sometimes books come along that we do not easily forget. When you read this book you will know why this is one of them. Congratulations to all the parents, the advisers and to Dr Anne Tracey for this life-changing book which must be required reading in every clinical setting, maternity facility, GP practice, HR office, fertility advice centre and in all the organisations that care for and support people through grief.

Dr Marie Murray, Editor; and Series Editor, *MindYourSelf*

ACKNOWLEDGEMENTS

It has been the greatest honour to bring this book to fruition and there are many people to thank.

First of all I would like to pay my respects to 'Kathy' and 'Leo', two contributors who sadly passed away before the book was completed. My thoughts are with their respective partners 'Ernest' and 'Gretta', and their families. I am thankful that permission was granted to include both testimonies yet sad too that they did not live to see their important insights in print.

Without the willingness of the courageous mums and dads who shared their tender stories of loss so openly and honestly, the book would not have been written. Deepest thanks to you all for your significant contributions and it is your voices that are at the core of each chapter, 'educating' us all.

I am forever grateful for the support of Dr Marie Murray, *MindYourSelf* Series Editor. Marie walked alongside me on the journey, and from the outset it was clear that the book was in kind and caring hands. I appreciate, beyond words, the gracious way in which Marie guided me through the process of bringing the chapters and the book to completion.

My thanks are also due to Cork University Press, especially Publications Director Mike Collins and Editor Maria O'Donovan, and to Aonghus Meaney and Alison Burns.

I feel blessed and owe a debt of gratitude to all of you who have offered endless support and encouragement along the way – I deeply appreciate it. Thank you from my heart.

My beloved Tracey family, John, Joel, Gayle and Órla. Gerry, thank you for the technical support that was essential for the interview recordings.

The Corey family in Moneymore (Jack and Phil, Brian, Desmond, Michael and Annette) and Long Island (Brendan and Pat) – the loss of our brother Patrick was the catalyst for this journey of learning, insight and healing. Remembering too our eldest brother Frank and his wife Monica who lived in Canada. Both deceased.

Eamonn Baker, for your belief in me and steadfast support throughout these past years.

Louise and John O'Donovan, Dublin and Marguerita and James McGovern, Galway for your kindness in allowing me to stay in your welcoming homes.

To all my dear and loyal friends, beautiful human beings that you are. I could not have been without your support and kindness on this journey.

I wish to acknowledge all those who helped to facilitate the process of the study:

Marie Cregan, University College Cork and Féileacáin

Staff at Galway University Hospital and Merlin Park University Hospital, Galway

Dr Geraldine Gaffney

Anne McKeown, Bereavement Officer/End of Life Care Committee

Colette Collins, Administrator, Clinical Research Ethics Committee

Assistant Professor Conor McGuckin, School of Education, Trinity College Dublin

Carole McKeeman, Bereavement Co-Ordinator, Western Health and Social Care Trust

Melissa Crockett, Childbirth and Loss Specialist Midwife, Western Health and Social Care Trust

Former colleagues and dear friends at Ulster University,

Magee Campus, Derry

My deepest thanks and appreciation are also due to:

My two colleagues, Fiona and Rosemary, at Yellow Wood Consultancy Ltd

Staff and friends at:

Macmillan Cancer Support

Physical Health Psychology Services, Altnagelvin Hospital

Foyle Hospice, Derry

Gestalt Institute of Ireland

My sincere thanks to Professor Assumpta Ryan, Professor of Ageing and Health, School of Nursing and Institute of Nursing and Health Research at Ulster University, for her support, encouragement and belief in this book.

INTRODUCTION

Dear Reader

First of all, welcome and thank you for choosing *Say My Baby's Name*. It occurs to me that a book on stillbirth and miscarriage would not be a topic readily selected from the shelves of a bookstore or ordered online. It is a book that may be sought out by bereaved mums or dads, like you, who 'know' what it is to experience the life-changing loss of a baby and who are drawn to the stories of those who share the same tragic loss. While your individual story may be different, you may identify with the experiences in the chapters ahead and feel as if you are reading about yourself! For some of you, the book could be an opportunity to understand the deeper meaning of the loss of a much-wanted baby if someone close to you has come through this difficult experience. Whatever your history, I hope and trust you will find solace and comfort in the stories shared so openly and honestly.

There is much to learn about losing a precious baby — at whatever stage of pregnancy the baby's life comes to an end — in the early stages, in the later stages, or close to the birth. As we will discover in the pages ahead, no matter when or at what stage the loss occurs, the pain is deeply felt; it takes a huge toll on the emotional, mental, physical and spiritual health of bereaved parents.

This book is based on one-to-one interviews with five men and twenty-seven women from across the island of Ireland. The thirty-two interviewees included four couples. At the time the study began in mid-2016, those who courageously volunteered to take part had suffered the loss of their baby through stillbirth or miscarriage within the previous ten years. It was important, however, that a minimum of two years had elapsed since the loss to ensure that taking part would not be detrimental to the emotional health and well-being of the interviewees.

In sharing their stories, twelve people spoke about the lived experience of loss through stillbirth and twenty about the lived experience of loss through miscarriage, which in some cases included multiple losses. In the first instance, we learn about the specific wish to have a baby or the surprise when a pregnancy was confirmed. Some were well resourced with family and a network of support, others less so. Some encountered miscarriage or stillbirth for the first time, others lived in fear of another loss.

Through their willingness to share their own losses, the interviewees have given us what is beyond price – the lived, raw reality of some of the most significant and most painful moments in their lives. There is no doubt that, for many of you, the poignant stories will be eye-opening and heart-opening, as you make your way through each of the chapters.

I am sure you are interested, as I was, in what motivated the men and women to come forward so willingly for the interviews. Not surprisingly, among other reasons, the study was seen as a way to speak – in many cases for the first time – about the loss that had impacted so profoundly.

It is these voices that speak to you now.

'Still my baby, still their heartbeat'

The person I am going to begin with is Tess. Her motivation to take part in the study and to share her experience with readers came from the loss of her daughter Leonie Ellen at full-term and two other babies in the early stages of pregnancy. She recounted with sadness a story of her husband's granny who 'never got to meet her baby boy'. Born without life, the baby was taken away in the boot of a car and buried. This tragic story led me to think of a friend who was denied the opportunity to see her baby. Family members thought they were doing the right thing and preventing more heartache by 'removing' and burying the baby. We know that this can only cause unspeakable pain that makes it more difficult for time to heal.

Tess feels that raising awareness is critical. Her key message is that no matter at what stage the loss happens, it is a loss and needs to be recognised and acknowledged:

> … it doesn't matter if it was eight weeks at the loss, it still is very much a loss. Still my baby, still their heartbeat.

Another interviewee, Tony, endorsed this view:

> … there are incredible definitions of stillbirth and miscarriage – certain number of weeks and timescales. I don't think it really matters to the parent.

Áine felt that if she communicated her experience, someone else might benefit: '… there has to be some good that comes out of it'.

Ruth agreed. She still feels the impact of the loss that needs to be spoken about:

> … it's nine years since I had a miscarriage and it's had such a big impact on my life. It's not spoken about and when I saw this opportunity to be interviewed, I thought I would like to speak about it. So that's why I am here today.

Leo, who was still grieving the loss of twins, was alerted to the study by his wife Gretta. However, Leo revealed that in the intervening ten years, as a couple they had *not* spoken to each other about the loss, although they did have a conversation in the car on the way to the interview. Leo welcomed the 'opportunity to talk'. Gretta too revealed that the interview was her first time to speak in-depth to anyone. She was supportive of the study that set out to encapsulate both men's and women's experiences of loss.

Having endured fourteen miscarriages and an ectopic pregnancy, Bridget holds that miscarriage is 'swept under the carpet'. She wanted to tell her story so that others could learn from her experience and was keen to remind us that the bereaved never forget: lost babies are eternally remembered, especially on significant days such as birthdays and Christmas.

Jane came along willingly but apprehensively. At the time, she wondered what questions might be asked and indeed if she would be able to recall her experience of loss. As it turned out, when Jane began to speak, her memories were, as she described them, 'very fresh'.

It is important to say that there were a number of other people who expressed an interest in taking part in the research. Some were 'outside' the framework of years that had been approved by ORECNI [Office for Research Ethics Committees Northern Ireland] and therefore could not be included but I hold their stories in my heart.

My personal story: growing up close to grief

You may be interested to know what has motivated the idea of an all-Ireland study of stillbirth and miscarriage. From the moment we are born our lives are shaped by everything that happens to us along the way, the choices we make and the opportunities that are afforded to us (or not). I grew up in a family that included my mam, Susan Corey, my dad, Frank Corey (both now deceased), and six lovely brothers: Frank (now deceased), Jack, Brendan, Brian, Desmond and Michael. Mam later told me she prayed for a girl during her final pregnancy and she got her wish. There was great delight when I arrived in the springtime of that year.

In their early lives, our parents suffered significant life-changing losses. Both of their mothers, Ellen Higgins and Margaret Corey, died when they were very young. Ellen died four days before Mam's seventh birthday and Margaret when Dad was fourteen. The deep feelings of sadness and grief of those earlier losses were retriggered for both our parents when their third son, Patrick, was stillborn at full term. Throughout the rest of her ninety years, Mam often referred to her 'dead born' son, a loss from which she never fully recovered. Patrick was born in an era when there was little opportunity to talk or be listened to. In those times, it seemed that grief and loss was silently endured.

In interviews with twelve women in Northern Ireland about their recollections of pregnancy loss in the 1940s, '50s and the beginning of the '60s, Rosanne Cecil found that the tragedy was rarely spoken about. The women 'struggled to make personal sense of their loss' and to understand why it had happened. '… nobody ever said we are sorry you lost your baby', one woman reported. Another said: '… that's fifty years ago, nobody ever talked about it'.

Growing up, I was naturally curious as to what had happened to my brother Patrick. In her life journey, profound grief had silenced Mam; the 'weight' of loss was visible, never far from the surface. Somehow, I managed to initiate a few 'intimate' conversations with her and learned that Patrick was alive and well late into the pregnancy. One day he was kicking ferociously in the womb, then the movements stopped. Mam felt that something was wrong and when Patrick was delivered two weeks later, it came to light that he had been strangulated by the umbilical cord. The Corey family was drenched in sorrow.

Patrick's little body was put into a white shoe-box. Our dad carried him to be laid to rest in the periphery of the graveyard at the local church. At the time, in the Catholic tradition, stillborn babies were not allowed to be buried in 'consecrated' ground. It is recognised within Catholicism that baptism is the sacrament that initiates children into the faith community. Therefore, for many generations, babies who died before baptism were not allowed funerals and could not be buried in church graveyards.

When my dear friend, the County Derry writer and poet Maura Johnston, was on sabbatical in Donegal completing her recently published book of poetry, *The Whetstone*, she felt compelled to write a poem ('Road's End') about Oileán na Marbh, the tiny island at Carrickfinn, County Donegal which translates as the 'Island of the Dead'. An estimated 500 stillborn babies, born mainly between the years of the Great Famine and 1912, were reportedly carried to the tiny island by night for secret burial, as they could not be buried on consecrated ground. Tragic losses within her own family motivated Maura to write the poem. Her mother miscarried a baby boy, christened Malachy, who was 'buried in a 2lb jampot'. Maura never knew where he was laid to rest. Later, her brother and sister-in-law's first two baby girls, Mary and Bridget, died in the womb. Maura recalled how she and her husband Kevin returned home from Africa when Bridget passed away: the baby was buried in a little hand-made box and the only people present were three family members. There was no input from the church.

In an arresting six lines, Maura creates a powerful image of the uneasy resting place at Oileán na Marbh:

The grey road stops at the sea
That rocks the Island of the Dead
Where the unclaimed and the unbaptised
Are abandoned to a gull-harsh rest,
restless as those rocking waves,
quiet as the hush of evening.

We might pause now and consider the turmoil that families must surely have felt in secretly burying their stillborn babies, shamefully hidden away because they were not entitled to a baptism, funeral or burial in consecrated ground. The pain of it all unseen, but nevertheless pain that families rarely escape from in their lifetimes.

In our family, we discovered that the main source of Mam's continuing worry, as a woman of faith, was that Patrick had not been baptised and would therefore not be in heaven. Determined to offer help and support, our brother Brian contacted the local priest. After years of fretting, Mam finally found the comfort and solace she needed when the priest visited and reassured her that Patrick would indeed have been baptised through 'baptism of the will': in other words, at the time of his birth, it would have been the wish and desire of our parents that their baby son was baptised, therefore through the 'will' he *was* baptised. We were all amazed at how quickly Mam seemed to relax, and how at ease she looked, now that her mind was lifted. We wish we had acted sooner.

Thankfully, since around 2007, wisdom and insight has brought about much-needed change in the Catholic Church's thinking regarding appropriate rituals for stillborn babies and those lost during pregnancy. Thankfully, too, we have recorded Patrick's name on the family grave that is now a source of solace and comfort to us all. It is the recognition and validation of our baby brother that is significant and gratifying, as is honouring our parents in the loss of their son. Perhaps some of you have had the same experience *and* the same drive to honour your history and legacy of loss. It is never too late to do so.

Waking up

I returned to education as a mature student, graduated in psychology and began an eight-year programme of supervised practice towards a chartership in psychology. I also became a volunteer counsellor with Foyle Cruse Bereavement Care. Later, having secured a post as a lecturer in the School of Psychology at Ulster University, it was imperative that I undertake doctoral research. What did I want to study and know more about? What were the gaps in research, especially in Ireland, that needed attention? In the end, it was the experiences that had shaped and influenced my life that I leaned towards.

Growing up 'close to grief', having personal experience of loss, gaining insights through psychology, and engaging in therapeutic work with many bereaved people drew my attention to areas of study that were closely associated with my life and my history. My first published work examined the psychological impact on daughters of the early loss of their mother; and now in this work, the privilege of unearthing men's and women's experiences of stillbirth and miscarriage.

Naturally, I was interested in what other research had been undertaken in Ireland and beyond. I discovered that many valuable books and papers on the subject of pregnancy loss had been published by various researchers including Rosanne Cecil (noted above), Bernadette McCreight, Aileen Mulvihill and Trish Walsh, among others. In a sense, I am now following in their footsteps and continuing the search for a deeper understanding of the impact of stillbirth and miscarriage.

The development of the book

I have been immersed in this work since 2016, while still teaching in the School of Psychology at Ulster University. The first step was to gain ethical permission. The study was initially approved by Ulster University Research Ethics Committee [UUREC] and then by the Office for Research Ethics Committees Northern Ireland.

In preparation for the book, I personally carried out, recorded, transcribed and analysed all of the one-to-one interviews that were undertaken at different locations across the island of Ireland. A tremendous feat, yet one that was cherished each step of the way. While it was and remains personally important to be inclusive and representative, the book has limitations. For example, I wanted to include those in same-sex relationships who had become pregnant and who had sadly lost their baby through stillbirth or miscarriage. A former student at Ulster, Laura Kennedy, provided an invaluable list of all LGBTQI organisations across Ireland. I made a huge effort through word of mouth and in correspondence with the different agencies to find a willing participant or participants. While the study was endorsed and welcomed, the search did not result in a volunteer being found. This remains a source of disappointment to me on their behalf. However, I can only hope that those who choose to read the book regardless of background, culture, religion or ethnic identity will find it helpful. Further research might focus on the testimonies of those who are not represented here.

I have been holding the stories of loss and a sense of this book in my head and heart since the study began. The stories shared sometimes made me shudder; made me think; made me cry; made me sit up and take notice; and confirmed unreservedly that this book is essential.

The best way to learn about these experiences is with the people who have endured the painful loss. Indeed, without the willingness of the thirty-two men and women involved, we would not be able to embark on this journey.

To ensure that as much insight as possible is gained through the shared experiences, the 'voices' of the bereaved parents remain central in the chapters. Where helpful, insights gained through research are included to endorse and support important messages. The reflections at the end of each chapter are intended partly as a summary and partly as an opportunity to pose further questions that may serve as food for thought. Importantly too, bereaved parents have key recommendations for change that they ask us all to consider. These are addressed in the Appendix:'Dialogue with Healthcare System'.

I hope that *Say My Baby's Name* will bring to the fore the breadth and depth of meaning attached to the life-changing loss of a much-wanted baby and will be of help to anyone who wishes to know more about the experience of stillbirth and miscarriage. Perhaps the experiences shared will help you feel less alone on your journey. The book may also help to enlighten and inform families and employers, as well as the medical and therapeutic professions who all too often encounter women and men bereaved of a baby.

It is important to stress to all our readers, and especially in deference to our medical colleagues, that we recognise that any references to or details of medical interventions or procedures contained in this book are the accounts articulated by participants and do not in any way constitute medical advice or guidance.

I wish you well as you begin to read the chapters ahead.

Anne

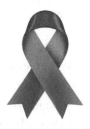

CHAPTER 1

'As soon as you know you are pregnant, the relationship begins'

Children are your little dreams that you put into this world,
hope incarnate ... people need hope ...

Willie

I t is well recognised that pregnancy and childbirth are hugely important and significant landmarks in the lives of parents. In the following pages you will hear the stories of many parents who learned that a baby was on the way. This discovery, not surprisingly, can be accompanied by a wave of emotions, which, as we will see, was the case for the parents in this book. As mums and dads cast their minds back, some relayed their memories with wistful smiles and even a little laughter; others were visibly sad as they spoke, no doubt mindful of the heart-rending grief that followed.

One of the key messages that came through in the accounts you are about to read is this: as soon as you know you are pregnant, the 'relationship' with the baby begins. Whether the news is met with shock, surprise or disbelief, there is a new relationship to be embraced from that moment on. Once those initial feelings subside, and reality sinks in, parents begin to focus on the future, the potential and the excitement that surrounds the arrival of new life.

We begin the stories in this chapter with Gabrielle, who summarised the developing relationship beautifully when she spoke of the 'joy, anticipation and wonder' of carrying a baby.

Gabrielle had lived a full life until the age of thirty-five and perceived herself to be an independent career woman with lots of freedom and lots of holidays. Like many women when they discover they are pregnant, a myriad of emotions descended upon Gabrielle all at once. Mixed in with the joy and excitement was the 'nervousness and apprehension' of a new journey, a new future life that was about to unfold. Even though a family holiday coincided with her news, Gabrielle was determined not to tell anyone until 'nearer the twelve-week mark'.

Another parent with a story to tell is Grace. Grace's life was somewhat complicated when she found herself to be pregnant again, as she was already a single parent. She described how her life had 'fallen apart' as 'the baby's daddy wasn't in the picture'. At the same time as the pregnancy began, Grace was diagnosed with depression. As she recounts it, she was not depressed at all, she was 'just pregnant again' and delighted with it. Grace believes that from conception it *is* a baby; a human being that you identify with and who creates great joy:

I started to identify with the baby and what it might look like and how it would feel to hold him and talk to him ... I was overjoyed ... I was going to be a mammy again and that was my hopes and my dreams and my plans. I had the vision of the nursery ... and a plan based around this ...

The intense feeling of 'relationship' was echoed by Maura, who spoke tenderly about the baby that was developing in her womb:

You are guarding and protecting that baby and you are nursing it to grow.

Many parents described the preparations they made and the future they imagined. As Grace indicated, the 'relationship' that is forming results in many preparations for the arrival of a newborn, as the various parents in this book describe:

• Tony and Betty 'bought all the bits and pieces needed' for Joshua.

23

- Drew and Jo decorated the baby's room, bought furniture and put Zach's name on the wall ready for the homecoming.

- Drew explained that a substantial amount of money was spent on prams and cots and 'everything needed' for Zach.

Drew recounted that he was away from home working in Holland and Belgium when a picture message arrived on his mobile phone. It looked like the results of a pregnancy test but he had to drive for a couple of hours before he could phone his wife Jo, who confirmed the good news. Referring to the picture message, Drew asked: 'Is that what I think it is?' And the joyful response came back: 'Yes, it is what you think it is!'

We can imagine the excitement and the thrill of that moment when the good news is shared. We also know that the moment of good news is in stark contrast to the moment when happiness turns into sorrow.

Maria and Archie wanted two children. Maria had a child from a previous relationship and decided to try for another baby. Just after Christmas both she and Archie were overjoyed at the news of a baby on the way. Eimear too recalled similar feelings. She knew that she wanted more children; however, the pregnancy came as a 'big, big surprise'. It wasn't planned but when it happened 'it was great'.

Planning, wanting and 'just needing' to get pregnant

Emily and John already had two daughters and Caoimhe was planned. While there was great excitement and delight all round, Emily noticed that she felt a little bit different 'this time', perhaps less excited that she did with the first two.

At the time, she did not really understand why.

Beth too planned her baby. She had been trying for a year but had to wait a little longer for the good news:

> I was quite young and so I kind of thought as soon as we started trying we would get pregnant.

The biological clock was ticking for Betty and she was feeling the pressure of 'just needing' to get pregnant. It happened very quickly in the end. Her husband Tony echoed his joy at the news:

> That's my son in there, that's my daughter in there … I'm going to be a dad!

Of course, as we know, pregnancy is met with a variety of emotions and not everyone receives the news with immediate delight. When researchers asked almost 5,000 women to recall the emotion/s they felt when their pregnancy was medically confirmed, it was noted that, among other factors, a planned pregnancy, the age of the parents and the level of social support seemed to generate a more positive outlook at the time and in the months ahead. However, as we are about to learn, the psychological impact of hearing this life-changing 'news' can evoke all kinds of different emotions in couples and within the wider family.

- Sometimes there is shock.

- Sometimes there is fear.

- Sometimes there is uncertainty.

People may also feel that they are too young, or too old, or not ready, or that the pregnancy is so unexpected that they cannot take in the reality just now.

'Shocked and scared'

Tara was 'shocked and scared' when she found out that she was pregnant, as the pregnancy was unplanned. She was living away from home at the time and had many thoughts 'swirling round' in her head.

Lilly was unsure when she discovered she was expecting Amilia Rose. She too was scared:

We were young, we only moved in to our wee house and you know when it's not planned it's a scary thing.

That she was in shock was an understatement when Ruth found out she was expecting her fifth child. But shock was soon followed by 'pure delight'. However, she never got to 'make the big announcement' to her husband as she was sick 'from three minutes in'. So he knew right away. However, in preparing for the arrival of her baby, Ruth was cautious in making her plans. She kept the pram and crib in the attic until they would be needed.

Sarrah, at forty-nine, thought, 'Surely not at my age.' At first, she could not understand the metallic taste in her mouth. Then she remembered that the only other time she experienced this was when she was pregnant with her daughter. She bought the 'most expensive pregnancy test' that quickly confirmed: 'pregnant: four weeks'. After that 'everything went into a tailspin'. First came shock. Sarrah initially did not want to believe that she was pregnant and had many questions:

How am I going to tell the children?

How am I going to afford to keep this child?

How can I work and watch the baby?

How can I work and afford childcare so that I can provide for the baby?

'I thought I would be sitting at seventy and my child is going to be twenty! The things that go through your head are nuts.'

But when Sarrah reached around twelve weeks, she and her daughter went to Mothercare and bought a wee suit to bring the baby home in. The preparations had begun.

It was a shock too for Mary when she heard she was pregnant. 'Our baby was eleven and I was turning forty. [I thought] I am going to be the oldest mother at the school gates.' But when the shock subsided, she started to enjoy it and 'get all excited'.

'Icing on the cake'

Confirmation that they were expecting twins was 'the icing on the cake' for Gretta and Leo, who already had children. Gretta recalled sitting in a car park outside a row of shops with her son and his friend. She was aware that she had been feeling tired and unwell, which prompted her to buy a pregnancy test. She 'could not believe' it when the result was positive; neither could her husband Leo, who immediately announced: 'Pregnant, brilliant … just get past the twelve weeks and we are on the road!'

When her relationship became more serious, Jane set parameters – marriage first and then children. Keen to have a baby with the wonderful man in her life, Jane wanted to be sure that there was commitment in the relationship. 'We got married,' she said. 'I stopped taking the pill and within a couple of months I was pregnant.'

Áine's pregnancy was 'a bit of good news' after the trauma of her husband's accident which left him significantly incapacitated for some time. When they started to get their life back on track and began to focus on having a family, Áine was delighted when she became pregnant 'almost straight away'. She very badly wanted to be pregnant at the time and went on to describe how it felt to 'connect' with the baby in the womb:

You imagine what the child is going to be like, what you are going to do together. I don't know anyone that gets pregnant and doesn't imagine …

Bridget's story was a little different. She was trialled on a fertility drug that, she says, 'kick starts your ovaries and controls your system'. She could not believe it that in the first month of the trial she became pregnant.

Kathy, who at the time was being treated for other health-related issues, questioned if the medication she was on could have affected her period, as it had not arrived when it should have. She was curious to know what was wrong. Following further health investigations, the nurse requested a urine sample. To Kathy's surprise, delight and shock, the nurse reported back: 'Congrats, you are pregnant!'

Reflection

The anticipation of a new life brings with it an avalanche of emotions. For some, there may be a period of emotional adjustment in coming to terms with the news. But let us not forget one of the significant threads running through these interviews – the 'relationship' with the baby that begins for almost every parent from the moment the news is confirmed.

Unlike previous generations, expectant mothers and fathers today could probably not imagine going through their pregnancy without an ultrasound scan. Advances in technology, introduced from the mid-1950s onwards, have increased our knowledge and understanding of the development of the growing embryo and perhaps contributed to a deepening of the relationship between parent and baby in the womb. Traditionally, the much-anticipated scans begin at around twelve weeks, followed by the twenty-week landmark, and beyond. It is understandable that when a much-wanted baby becomes visible on the screen, it makes the new life that is forming more 'real' for both mum and dad – this *is* their child, a human being with a heartbeat, growing and developing, waiting to be born. The introduction of scanning has provided the welcome opportunity for fathers to be 'included' in the journey through pregnancy – it is their child too. We can hear the excitement and joy in Tony's words: '… that's my son in there, that's my daughter in there … I'm going to be a dad!'

So, the accounts in this chapter hold a very important message for us all. The news of a pregnancy – whether it is expected or unexpected; whether it is a shock and/or a surprise; planned or unplanned – is the beginning of a very special journey in life. With the news comes the hopes and as-pirations which are foremost in the minds of most expectant parents as they begin to imagine the future and what it might hold for their child. The enormity then of discovering that all is not well in the pregnancy is what we need to respond to with compassion and empathy. In the next two chapters we learn more about the impact of that news, which brings such devastation, grief and loss.

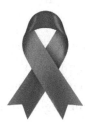

CHAPTER 2

'Something was wrong'

The consultant said the foetus isn't thriving ...

Jane

The accounts in the previous chapter offer us an important reminder of how significant the news of a pregnancy can be. We learned also that whether planned or unplanned, 'attachment' to the new life begins from the moment the news breaks.

However, the joy of the pregnancy news was, for some parents, short-lived. The anticipation of a new baby coming into the family was overshadowed by worry and concern when, in the early months, something began to feel 'not quite right' or there were signs that 'something was wrong'.

In this and the next chapter, mums and dads poignantly describe, in some detail, first their experience of learning that all was not well, and then their memories of losing their baby. Sometimes, indicators were there but the overwhelming hope that everything would be fine meant that it was difficult to acknowledge 'signs', and so these may not always have been taken on board. All experiences are unique and yet there are similarities in the stories.

We learn how mums and dads tried to manage the devastating signs that their pregnancy was at risk. Parents also shared memories of interactions with consultants, doctors and midwives who broke the news. Some went beyond the diagnosis or set of symptoms to support and empathise; others did not. We know that the way in which medics convey the news is forever remembered and the impact can be far-reaching. Through interviews with eight women in the west of Ireland who had experienced the loss of their baby, researchers

Aileen Mulvihill and Trish Walsh highlighted the importance of medical professionals engaging in honest and sensitive communication with bereaved parents as emotional reactions are exacerbated when there is a lack of appreciation of the loss.

Perhaps some of you engaging with these often hard to read accounts will resonate with the heartfelt experiences that are shared. We turn first to Jane, whose poignant story helps us to understand how difficult it is to absorb the distressing news.

'I carried on about my business'

Jane was tearful as she recalled the moment she heard the news, ten weeks into her pregnancy, that her baby was not going to survive. She remembered how the consultant was kind and considerate when he told her that the 'foetus wasn't thriving'. Jane had just transferred into a new post at work and as she was pregnant she volunteered to be the designated driver at the Christmas 'do'. However, when she arrived at the venue she noticed 'a wee spot of blood', a new development that concerned her greatly. As the days passed, the spotting got heavier. Having been sent for an ultrasound of her kidneys, Jane made the radiographer aware that she was around ten weeks pregnant, to which there was no response! Jane 'didn't twig that anything was wrong', she 'carried on about her business'. During her next visit, the GP consulted a letter that had arrived from the hospital and asked: 'Could your dates be wrong?' This was the start of coming to terms with the sad news.

The experience for Betty was somewhat different. In the department where she worked at the time, she explained, there were three other women pregnant. Everyone was commenting on how 'neat' and 'small' Betty's 'bump' was compared to the others'. At the time she 'felt like a whale' so she did not pay too much attention to the remarks.

Whatever the circumstances that bring about the end of a pregnancy, there are certain occurrences that by definition make the situation more traumatic than it might otherwise be. Most stark, shocking and traumatic perhaps are the devastating situations when a baby ends up in a toilet bowl. The imagery, the significance. As we listen to the mothers speak frankly about the shock and trauma of their baby ending up like this and the horrendous sense of loss and grief they experienced in having to flush their baby away, we become conscious of the enormous tragedy for every parent who has lost a child, at whatever stage of gestation that may be. There is a fierce need to retain the dignity of these little beings and what happens when viability ends.

The remainder of this chapter may be tough to read. You may not be able to continue and may need to pause and come back later. However, it is important to share and honour the poignant histories so that we can understand fully the difficult emotional journey that parents endured.

Before continuing to the next section, I feel the need to discuss the meaning of trauma, and what I have learned about trauma through the teachings of psychotherapist and trauma specialist Bríd Keenan. Trauma creates within the person a disconnection from self and other, including a disconnect from emotions and the physical body. As a result, it can be difficult to live in the present moment, but one way to begin the process of healing and recovery is through 'body work', known as somatic experiencing – a type of therapy that focuses on the connection between the mind and body.

Through this approach recovery means:

- reconnecting with the body
- reconnecting with the emotions
- reconnecting with the self
- reconnecting with other.

Recovery from trauma is possible. However, when trauma remains unresolved, it continues to live on in the body and will manifest itself in the form of various ailments over the longer term.

'Everything came out in the toilet bowl'

It was confirmed when Catherine was eleven weeks pregnant that she was miscarrying. She and her partner were sitting in the waiting area of the hospital where nurses were discussing the best places to hang up some newly acquired artwork for the ward. She vividly recalled speaking sharply to the nurse at the desk: 'Could you hurry up and see me; I'm sitting here bleeding, I'm losing my baby.'

When an examination confirmed what she feared, in a state of devastation Catherine had to face back out to where pregnant women were sitting, waiting to be seen:

With tears rolling down my face I nodded to my partner and burst into tears; they quickly ushered me into another room where I got myself together. I could see the pity of the other women as I left the ward. I was sent home and told to return if I began to cramp or the bleeding got heavier. I went to bed early and managed to sleep, probably exhausted from crying. The next morning, I woke up covered in blood from the waist to the knees. When I got up to the bathroom I got the feeling that I was trying to hold something in. Everything came out into the toilet bowl, loads of clots, blood, dark stuff; my baby down the toilet. It was very traumatic and I was in shock.

Grace worried too that her baby had 'gone down the toilet'. She was in bed for a long time and knew that she was losing her baby. She felt able to 'pinpoint the moment' when there was no life anymore. She had been sleeping and woke up with the thought 'the baby is away'. To think that her baby had gone down the toilet was 'extremely upsetting'. However, Grace's mother came to the rescue: she held the view that if the baby had gone down the toilet, then he or she had gone into the river, then into the sea and was part of the cycle of life – this was a concept that Grace found comforting and helpful.

Having had four healthy pregnancies with no problems, Ruth expected that her latest would be the same. When she started spotting it was 'a complete and utter shock'. Within days she started bleeding heavily, and cramping. When Ruth and her husband arrived at the hospital for help and support she became unwell and had to rush to the toilet:

I had been given a dish in case I passed anything. I had the miscarriage into the dish in the toilets of accident and emergency. A roar came out of me that I have never heard before and I hope I never hear again … my own voice … it just came out of me very naturally. And my husband rushed to the door and came in; we didn't know what to do then.

I didn't think it was appropriate to flush away my baby that was now in a dish.

As she waited for further examination, Ruth knew her baby was still in the tray in the bathroom she had just left. She asked a nurse who passed by about her baby and was told not to worry, it would be sorted. Some time later, while still waiting, she asked again about her baby and was told: 'It's gone.'

Let us pause here and say that this is not a decision for a health professional to make, however well intentioned it may appear to be. Psychology has become increasingly aware of the importance of respect and ritual, naming and burying even at very early gestational stages, because for parents this is the loss of their 'baby'.

'It all feels very surreal ...'

Beth described herself as always being conscious of her body. She had 'erratic and strange periods' and the doctor suspected cysts at one point. Eleven weeks into her pregnancy (just ten days before her first scan was due) Beth knew that 'something felt really strange' even though she was not sick or unwell per se. But things changed very quickly as early-morning spotting changed to heavy bleeding by the end of the day. Despite her own doctor's advice to 'rest and wait at home' given that she was not having physical symptoms or sharp pains, a nurse in the family, seeing Beth distraught and in discomfort, took her straight to hospital. As Beth's doctor had predicted, there was nothing they could do. Beth was sent home with paracetamol and invited to come back in the next day for a scan:

I went home and it all feels very surreal now thinking about it … I was passing clots and I was looking at them because I was trying to figure out what was going on and at one point I thought there was a little tiny '*bean shape*' and … I became really distraught and said I just know that was my baby …

While her husband was unsure if it was possible to 'see' a baby in the early stages, Beth, having been used to passing large clots during periods, was sure that this passing was different from anything she had experienced before. The next day came the shattering news from the doctor, delivered with little clemency: 'The pregnancy test came back negative so you are not pregnant anymore.' Parents would welcome a review of how health professionals relate such important, often devastating, news. The concept of 'walk a mile in my shoes' comes to mind.

Let us pause again for a moment and say something about medical training. We know that medicine (as with psychology) is taught as a science. The qualified doctor is trained to be impartial when making a diagnosis based on the physical symptoms presented. While this is undoubtedly the case, a pregnant mother who is deeply concerned about the health and well-being of the baby she is carrying will be overcome by many emotions, including worry, fear, anxiety and fretfulness. Perhaps we could also speculate that the health professional's response is influenced by personality and personal life experience? Similarly, how the medic's response is perceived is determined by the expectations of the mother-to-be. Importantly, Bernadette McCreight, lecturer in the School of Sociology and Applied Social Studies in Ulster University and expert on the topic of perinatal loss, reminds us: 'Pregnancy loss is more than a medical experience and the way in which the event of a baby's death, whether by miscarriage or stillbirth, is socially constructed and acknowledged is crucial in helping women to come to terms with their grief.'

It was Valentine's Day, a day that Sarrah described as 'just another Saturday' but she did not know that life was to change in the early hours of the following morning. During those first twelve weeks she had 'wee smears' of blood but no pain. Sarrah regarded this as quite common as she had cervical erosion. Having the same symptoms in this pregnancy as she had previously with her daughter, Sarrah was convinced she was going to have a baby girl. She was waiting to get beyond the twelve-week 'danger point' before sharing the news. But then tragedy struck:

I went to bed that night and I woke with lower abdominal pains and pains in my back. Coming round from sleep I was sore and I very quickly realised that I was bleeding ... I was alone and it was dark ... my head's going all over the place because I realised I was losing the baby ... I could see the baby at the bottom of the toilet bowl ... a sort of purple-grey colour – and I know this sounds stupid but I was really shocked by the fact that she was so baby-shaped for being only twelve weeks. I wanted to lift her out and hold her and I was actually scared I would break her if I touched her. I had lost her, I wasn't able to protect her ... I just sat in the bathroom, just crying and looking ... And the worst thing of all was that I had to flush her away and I didn't want to do that.

We need to pause and try to digest the depth of pain in such a situation; and the helplessness and hopelessness felt in that moment where there are few options but to flush a precious baby away. We need also to think about burial rituals. If the loss of a baby at any gestational stage brings grief, then the rituals of bereavement should, perhaps, surround it. The accounts of these parents confirm the importance of that.

'I knew in my heart of hearts ...'

Áine knew something was not quite right. She went immediately to accident and emergency (A&E) when she began bleeding at around twelve weeks. While the nurse tried to instil hope, Áine knew in her 'heart of hearts' it was not good. She was invited to come back the next day to the early pregnancy unit (EPU), where she was scanned. The question arose: 'Are you sure your dates are right?'

The long-awaited honeymoon planned by Áine and her husband was cancelled. She tried to manage the painful cramps that followed without paracetamol, thinking she would prefer to be without them 'in case there was a baby still there'. Áine outlined the traumatic events of her loss:

> I got through really bad cramps up until about eleven at night. I went to sleep, and at ten to two I woke up again in excruciating pain. It was horrendous, I never felt pain like it in my life ... it felt like labour, like my whole body was contracting and ... it was starting and stopping. By this stage I was passing an awful lot of blood. There were clots in the blood ... It got so bad that I was bent over double

in the bathroom … My husband said, 'Listen, we are going straight to A&E.' It was horrendous.

Amy was sitting at home one night when she began to experience 'awful' stomach pain. She was kept in hospital for three nights as the scans were inconclusive and there was some thought that it could be an ectopic pregnancy. In the end, it was a miscarriage at eight weeks. The next pregnancy happened soon after and Amy got to nine or ten weeks and miscarried again.

Reflection

The heartfelt accounts in this chapter give a sense of the devastation felt by those trying to absorb the news that their baby's life is compromised. Christina Lee and Ingrid Rowlands of the University of Queensland interviewed nine Australian women who had suffered miscarriage and were told of the overwhelming emotions the women experienced and how they struggled to make sense of the loss of the pregnancy and 'the hope and dreams attached to this imagined life'.

We need to remember that for those who endure it, the loss of a baby can lead to anxiety, depression, low self-esteem, guilt and anger; and for some it can be the most traumatic event of their lives. Recovery is a long and lengthy process and many women remain emotionally affected for years afterwards.

Therefore, it would be remiss of us to underestimate the toll that the loss of a baby through miscarriage takes on parents' physical, mental and psychological health.

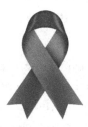

CHAPTER 3

'I am sorry, I cannot get a heartbeat'

A family's life and a couple's whole world just destroyed there in an instant …

Bridget

In this chapter we learn of the experiences of those who were faced with news that no parent wants to hear. We hear about the overwhelming shock and trauma that engulfs parents when they discover, particularly at a later stage in the pregnancy, that their baby has died. This experience inevitably ignites emotions of confusion, fear, distress and disbelief. And the manner in which it emerges that 'all is not well' plays a part in this: including where, when and how the information is conveyed, by whom and the degree to which sensitivity and awareness are present. There are crucial elements in the relating of traumatic news which, if mishandled or misunderstood by professionals, can affect people forever.

The devastating news can arrive suddenly and unexpectedly, like a bolt out of the blue. Some had 'warnings' that there were complications; at the end stage of pregnancy, others came to the sad realisation the baby's heartbeat could not be found. That realisation 'hits hard'. The world of expectant parents, as Bridget said, 'is destroyed in an instant'.

Psychological research on suffering and loss has always recognised the impact of hearing sad news and the significance of the moment and its aftermath. Parents are in shock, in disbelief; they are numb, confused, and may lose all sense of self; such is the human response, there may be a sensation or feeling of being out of body looking down on yourself. The detailed, sensitive and deeply moving accounts you are about to read provide acute insights into the lived experience of those who are told that their baby will be born without life or breath.

'This is not routine anymore'

Jo and Drew were faced with the trauma that their baby Zach would be born without life. As soon as the doctor put the Doppler on, Drew knew that he should hear the heartbeat or the gushing of the amniotic fluid surrounding baby Zach. He had seen it done before so he knew what to expect. But alarm bells started going off when there was complete silence. In his own mind, Drew frantically searched for reasons as the tragedy of the loss unfolded:

The Doppler [ultrasound used to monitor high-risk pregnancies] looked a bit different from the one I had seen before so maybe this is a different system ... all of these possibilities going on in my head and then the midwife said: 'Och he must have turned round, he is lying to the back, maybe I'll go and get another scanner ...

Drew continued:

So the big scanner comes in and starts to go for maybe ten minutes or so and the whole time Jo just looked at the ceiling – she knew! Still in my mind I wasn't sure ... the midwife left again and they brought in another scanner ... there's two doctors and three midwives in this little room. This is not routine anymore. They brought in the senior consultant, who continued to do the scan ... absolute silence … after about half an hour they said, 'There's no heartbeat … About thirty-six hours earlier we had been told happy healthy baby and then it is just gone as quickly as that. You don't see it happening …

Thirty minutes after they learned that Zach had died, Drew and Jo were told to go home. In their minds, it seemed unusual to be sent home so quickly after receiving such devastating news. Although most of their care was excellent, both were aware that an assessment had not been carried out on how they might cope with such a shock. To not be assessed or offered any information was considered a gap in their care at this critical stage. Literally they were told to come back the next morning.

This raised questions in Drew's mind as no one really checked if he was okay. No one knew how they were going to cope. So the question arises: what about emotional support for parents who have received the most traumatic news that their baby has died?

'It was like an out-of-body experience … we were in total disbelief'

Tess's story bears some similarities. Having experienced two miscarriages with babies Leo and Dylan, she was delighted that there were no major problems or complications in her pregnancy with Leonie Ellen. She attended all check-ups and everything was fine. Having seen the midwife on the 2nd of December, everything was in place and she was to be induced on the 9th. However, labour began two days earlier on the 7th.

When Tess arrived at the hospital after a painful start to the day (which she considered to be labour pains), the midwife observed that she looked 'very white'. As well as checking for infection, the midwife put on the monitor. Tess remembered in that moment that she did not hear a heartbeat. Her husband attempted to comfort her but when the midwife returned and put on the monitor again, baby Leonie's heartbeat could not be found. The midwife got the doctor to check. Tess said:

It was like an out-of-body experience … I was the person looking at me lying on the bed, thinking, *what is this person on about?* Almost like you are hallucinating; they are not talking to you about you. The doctor came along and said: 'Maybe the scanner is not working, we will get another one.'

Within minutes the doctor confirmed that there was no heartbeat.

I looked at the screen in disbelief and it felt like he wasn't talking about me, that he was delusional or something … at this stage we had no indication of what had happened; everything six days before had been fine. We were in total disbelief why this happened or how it could have happened.

Parents – fathers and mothers – are in the happy state of expecting a healthy baby to arrive, and in a moment their dreams are shattered. The shock, distress and trauma of the news is almost too much to bear.

'Maybe it's a quiet day for the baby'

Anna and Paul suffered this trauma. Anna was thirty-two weeks into her pregnancy with baby Gerry when she noticed something was not right. She alerted her husband Paul that she had not felt the baby move that day. It was summertime and Anna and her family were busy renovating the house. Compared to earlier pregnancies where she experienced 'crazy kicking', this baby was not overly active. She said: 'We just thought it was maybe a quiet day for the baby.' Normally ice cubes would 'stir on a wee bit of movement' but this time no movement. Anna questioned: 'How did I not notice?'

Anna realised that she could not go to a family wedding the following day without getting checked out first. She assumed the medics would just send her 'skipping away' so that she could happily attend the wedding.

Paul accompanied Anna to the hospital. Sadly, after a strenuous effort on the part of the medical team, the baby's heartbeat could not be found. Anna remembered:

> The wee nurse, the look on her face because she just could not find a heartbeat … They brought in a junior doctor … you could just see she wasn't experienced … it's just that realisation that they can't find anything … all that day I had felt no movement. To be honest I knew myself … this wasn't good.

When the consultant came in Anna became 'nearly hysterical'; she knew that it was true, and that it would be confirmed that her baby had died.

'Try harder … get someone else …'

Tony was in desperation when the consultant, who had been summoned, confirmed: 'I am sorry, I cannot get a heartbeat.'

Baby Joshua's heart had stopped beating. Tony broke down and pleaded:

> Try harder, get someone else … who is the next person? Get the new machine …

At this stage, Tony's wife Betty was forty weeks and five days into her pregnancy. When she reported reduced movement, the hospital advised her to take some cold water, lie down and see if anything happened. Betty had been cleaning the house from top to bottom that day and, being busy, had not noticed anything. She'd diligently attended all the six-weekly appointments under the care of the midwife. Everything was fine: she was measuring as she should and the heartbeat was always there. The first time she became aware there was a problem was on arrival at A&E. Apart from the tears and anguish, Betty and Tony do not remember much else after hearing the devastating news that Joshua had died.

'Alarm bells went off'

At the foetal assessment unit (FAU) when Mary was around eight or nine weeks pregnant her baby's heartbeat could not be found, but a number of weeks later a faint heartbeat did eventually register. At eighteen/nineteen weeks a bigger scan caused concern as the medics could not get baby Emmet Pio to move. When Mary was seen by the head consultant, 'alarm bells went off'. She studied the consultant's face as she observed the scan:

I just knew by the look on her face that she didn't like what she was seeing ... she told us to be prepared for some kind of diagnosis.

'I had no signs or symptoms'

At a check-up in the health centre, the midwife examined Maura with the Doppler (ultrasound) but could not find Ronan's heartbeat. It did not register with Maura that there could be something wrong. She had other children at home, including a baby. Following a recommended visit to her GP, who carried out a second scan, it was sad news. Maura explained:

> ... the wee baby was just lying still. I had no signs or symptoms – nothing. I was eighteen weeks ...

'This baby was coming at twenty-two weeks ...'

Kathy carried four boys – baby Hyam to twenty-two weeks, baby Solomon to eighteen weeks, baby Hezekiah to sixteen weeks and baby John to eleven weeks. With Hyam, the hospital said there was nothing they could do – 'this baby was coming at twenty-two weeks'. Kathy explained:

> They tested to see if there was a heartbeat after he was born because he was fully formed ... there was no heartbeat ... he was very long and he looked just like me and his eyes were open which was really strange for twenty-two weeks old ...

With Solomon it was recommended that a stitch (an intervention to prevent miscarriage, also termed cervical cerclage or cervical stitch) be put in. However, as she had other health complications and was attending two hospitals, Kathy passed the fourteen-week point at which the stitch should have been inserted, something she deeply regretted. The need for a stitch was not overlooked by a very vigilant consultant who looked after Kathy in her fifth pregnancy. With the insertion of a stitch at fourteen weeks, a healthy baby daughter arrived at thirty-seven weeks, much to the joy of Kathy and Ernest.

'I was in a bubble, completely numb … shell-shocked'

Waking up one morning with no movement, Rose rang the hospital. She was advised to eat some chocolate and move around. When this failed to make a difference, Rose's husband dropped her to A&E (as he had also done two days previously for her check-up).

Deep down, Rose knew that when two midwives – one after the other – scanned her and could not find a heartbeat, something was wrong. But it did not quite sink in. When a young doctor arrived and confirmed that Ellen's heartbeat could not be found, Rose remembered that he did so without any eye contact whatsoever:

And that was it … I didn't cry, didn't do anything. I felt like I was in a bubble – completely numb. Gerard [Rose's husband] came down and I was still in a cubicle … they told me I could go home or I could be admitted, and asked did I still want to have a section or they could give me a tablet to bring on labour. We didn't know what to do because we were still shell-shocked.

Importantly, the investigation that followed Ellen's stillbirth resulted in a written apology *and* a number of recommendations for the future care of pregnant women in Ireland. The report stipulated that when a mother with reduced movements comes in to get checked, a number of steps need to be followed. If it is not a first pregnancy, the case has to be reviewed by a consultant and patients should not be seen for clinical review without their full medical record to hand.

'She hasn't moved today …'

Lilly had a busy working life. In the middle of a work day she suddenly thought: *Oh, she hasn't moved today, Amilia Rose definitely has not moved.*

Lilly felt tired and decided to go home and lie down. It occurred to her that maybe Amilia could be sleeping. However, Lilly felt sick and recalled that 'something wafted over' her. Deep down she knew something was wrong. The hospital advised her to drink a glass of cold water, lie down and call back in an hour. Sadly, nothing changed. Lilly made the decision to drive herself to the hospital and not alert David, her husband. However, for some reason David left work early that day and was on his way home. When they met on the road, Lilly explained her concern. From there they drove to the hospital together in rainfall so heavy that visibility was drastically reduced.

The midwife who had taken Lilly's earlier phone call tried to find a heartbeat. Reassuringly, she advised not to panic as sometimes the baby's back can be at the front and heartbeat cannot be detected when that is the case. But Lilly knew Amilia was dead. What made a traumatic situation even more difficult was that the doctor on call was quite abrupt. This brings to the fore the plea by lecturer and expert on perinatal loss Bernadette McCreight. She asks that medical personnel be mindful of the status of the lost baby and of the fact that 'many women conceptualise their baby as an extension of their own being, a potential for lived life'.

'I never had doubts … that we weren't going to full term'

Leo and Gretta already had children when they joyfully discovered that a baby was on the way. The 'icing on the cake' was the news that it was twins. Sadly, after a few months, a scan revealed that one of the twins, later called Daniel, was no longer there. Gretta explained:

> The consultant referred to a ghost twin … there are definitely two there and then one disappears … it's absorbed back into the body …

Later in her pregnancy, while Gretta was visiting her father who was in hospital, she got worried:

> As I was sitting in the room with him I hadn't felt any movement and there was a stillness that I just knew there was something wrong. I didn't say anything to anybody.

Gretta chose not to share her concerns with anyone until she was sure of what was happening. Two days after her father died, Gretta went to maternity and got scanned. In her mind she was twenty weeks pregnant. The doctor said: 'I am really sorry, there is just no movement there.' The second twin, named Francis, had also died. This devastating news was difficult for Leo to accept. With a resounding heaviness, he explained his way of looking at it:

> I never had doubts in my mind at any stage that we weren't going to go full term … because we had been there twice before and you think there is nothing going to happen. So, you look forward to your third child …

Emily and John went for the twenty weeks scan very excited. At one point the midwife, whom they found to be very capable, 'stalled' and left the room to look for another medic. The anxiety in the room in that moment was almost palpable. Emily recalled John's words to her as they waited for the midwife to return:

> John said: 'What is going on? … there is something wrong … she didn't leave the room for no reason … just prepare ourselves for something coming.'

Reflection

Can we even begin to fathom what it must be like for any of those mothers and fathers who have spoken to us so courageously in this chapter? If we could, would we not be 'shell-shocked' too? Surely it is impossible to read the heart-rending accounts above and not feel deeply for those who have endured such a traumatic journey.

We have learned that when a couple hears that problems have arisen in the pregnancy, how they hear it, from whom, and the level of care and aftercare (if any) they receive has a significant psychological impact and can leave an enduring imprint. It is often assumed that because a couple have the support of each other, they will be fine. Drew's question – about emotional support for parents who have received the most traumatic news that their baby has died – deserves further consideration.

It is important to note that when miscarriage and stillbirth happen, anxiety and depression may follow for both mum and dad. Silence does not work. The key to counteracting any such mental health difficulties that might arise is talking, as well as solid support from family, the medical and therapeutic professions, support groups and employers.

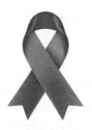

CHAPTER 4

'My body was screaming "baby"'

*It is difficult grieving a baby but wanting another baby ... you
are planning the next one in your head ... until I have a baby
in my arms screaming and crying I'll not be content.*

Tess

With five unforgettable, emotive words, 'My body
was screaming "baby"', Grace gave voice to the
physical, mental and emotional strain left behind
in the aftermath of the loss. As her words rang out in the
interview I could feel an ache rise inside of me, a mix of deep
empathy and sadness. Perhaps, reading this, you may feel
it now too. Distraught with grief that she described as 'all-
consuming and powerful', Grace could not accept that she
had lost her baby, as 'all the hormones and preparation had
started'.

Also, reading Tess's heart-rending desire for another baby
(above) makes us wonder what it must be like for mothers and
fathers, grieving the loss of their baby yet desperately wanting
another baby?

The insights in this chapter will help us understand that
longing to be pregnant again – even while still in the delivery
room! While the desire for a baby is acute, mothers remain
in a state of 'high alert' as they enter the emotional landscape
that comes with a new pregnancy. The previous loss will not
allow for complacency, or an assumption that all will be well.
The pregnancy is accompanied by a very real fear – that the
same thing will happen again. Each little step is carefully
monitored, on a daily basis. Emotions are raw and there is a
sense of vulnerability that was not present before. Nothing is
taken for granted.

We turn to Betty first, who reminds us that a 'rainbow' pregnancy – a pregnancy that follows a loss – is less joyful. 'It is nine months full of worry and anxiety; another baby does not "fix" things as there will always be something missing, a "hole" that cannot be filled.' Rose confirmed that the next pregnancy is like being in a bubble but it is '… less a bubble of joy, more one of anxiety and worry'.

Fathers are coping with their own despair and distress but often their attention turns to the health and well-being of their partner. In being strong and supportive, men are often taking on the role that culture demands of them. However, their true feelings can remain hidden and unsupported. Tony affirmed that '… most parents who lose a first baby want to have another one straight afterwards …'. In their determination to have another baby, Tony and Betty sought the help of a clinical psychologist to get back on track. Betty confirmed that there was no desire to replace Joshua, it was a deep-seated desire to have a baby in their life:

> Even in the delivery suite I was saying to myself I want to get pregnant again straight away … even though I couldn't even comprehend doing that … I felt like something needed to be replaced; not replaced – we were missing our baby and so we did try again …

When her new daughter arrived, Betty wondered if she had dealt fully with the loss of Joshua. In the first three to six months she found it impossible to comfort her baby girl. The struggle for Betty was to find a 'connection' and to overcome the feeling that she 'couldn't do anything right':

I felt like I had lost the opportunity to make that connection or that bond because when he [Joshua] was born there was that mad rush ... you are in love with your baby and it's all lovely emotions – it was the happiest and the saddest day in my life, all in the one day. When she was born I didn't feel that – she had been taken away to make sure she was breathing properly so I didn't get that immediate connection and this was followed by a difficult six months of being at home with her. I kind of felt like I had missed that chance to make the bond.

Betty has courageously raised a significant and important issue about becoming a mother while still grieving. Is the 'connection' with a new baby interrupted by the residue of grief for the lost baby? When a baby is taken away straight after the birth does that 'interrupt' the bonding process between mother and baby that is so important in those first few moments?

Losing a much-wanted baby, setting your heart on becoming pregnant again and discovering that you are pregnant is, to say the least, an emotional rollercoaster. Grace said it did not 'cure the problem' as she was still reeling from the loss:

My body might have been satisfied that there was a baby there but emotionally it was terrible ... I was bouncing around emotionally.

This points to a major issue, as it is hard for parents to say how much they want another baby without this being misinterpreted as disregard for the child they have lost. Of course it is not that at all, because every baby lost is a baby loved and mourned – but there is a deep-seated need to be pregnant, to fill the emptiness and ache left by the loss of a child. This was very true for Rose.

'The longing … is all-consuming'

Rose spoke of 'the longing' she felt to be pregnant again as 'all-consuming', and was clear that it had nothing to do with a desire to 'replace' Ellen:

It wasn't in any way to replace her … I just had this urge … this longing to hold a baby and straight away I was like we need to try again. It is mad. We went back to see the doctor … and he said, you have to be able for it emotionally. If you feel you are I will help you but you have to be ready.

That longing, Rose felt, interfered with the grieving process for Ellen as she had not fully grieved her baby daughter when she became pregnant again.

'A total rollercoaster …'

Tess's daughter Leonie Ellen was stillborn and then she suffered the loss of two babies, Leo and Dylan, through miscarriage. Tess, pregnant again at the time of the interview, helped us understand the complexities of the aftermath of loss:

It is difficult grieving a baby but wanting another baby. You have that loss, that emptiness … home feels very empty, very lonely. Then there is the physical side … it is a woman who goes through it and you have different feelings and emotions. With grief, part of you wants to be comforted, the other part of you doesn't want anyone near you. Trying for another baby when dealing with your loss is just a total rollercoaster. You want it to happen the first time, you want everything to go smoothly, you have a fear that it may happen again.

Tess added:

Until I have a baby in my arms screaming and crying I'll not be content … in your mind you are grieving this baby but you are planning the next one in your head. It does become an obsession … at thirty-three I am thinking I need to have a baby, I need to get pregnant. And then I became pregnant quite quickly.

When Anna got home from the hospital all she wanted to do was get pregnant. 'That's the God's honest truth,' she said. 'You want another baby.'

The loss of baby Gerry left Anna thinking she was moving on in age; she did not want to delay so she had her next two children in quick succession. But the loss of Gerry changed her outlook and made her more aware of not taking anything for granted:

Just because you get pregnant there is no guarantee you are going to have a healthy baby – there is some realisation in that. You think when you are pregnant that you will be coming out of the hospital with a baby that is alive and kicking and reality is just not the same.

'I couldn't think of anything else other than a second baby ...'

Bernadette agreed that after a miscarriage there is anxiety, particularly if it is a first baby. As others found, while the next pregnancy is welcome, it is hard to relax, there is constant worry. To alleviate the anxiety, Bernadette's GP sent her to the early pregnancy unit to get scanned and all was well.

Bernadette 'spent a fortune on hormone testing' as she 'couldn't think of anything else other than a second baby'. However, that total focus and attention seemed to come with a price:

> I was conflicted with guilt then as well because I had a beautiful boy who was growing up in front of me and I felt so guilty. I felt like I was just distracted from him all the time. But the logic between your head and your heart is just two totally different things. And I felt good when we were going through the treatment as I thought I am being practical – doing something practical.

Bernadette, however, described the arrival of her last baby, a little girl, as 'the cherry on top of our cake'. After the heart-breaking loss of the baby she was expecting at the time of the interview, she feels very lucky to have a beautiful new daughter in the family.

'Desperation turned into determination'

Catherine's experience resonated with the state of alertness that Bernadette spoke about:

Once you have had a miscarriage – every single time you go to the toilet you are checking yourself, you are on high alert; every little twinge is a worry – you are super-connected to your own body.

Catherine's reason for wanting to be pregnant was to give her child a sibling. She described in detail the drive and energy invested in her plan for another baby:

I was desperate to have another child and this nearly split us up; I knew I was not complete without another child. Desperation turned into determination. I had negativity in my life from earlier years and I thought I will make this work somewhere in my life. I was dogged that it was not going to control the rest of my life. I used hurt and anger to drive me; I was like a woman possessed ...

Catherine admitted that when she found out she was 'expecting again', both she and her husband Willie were 'on tenterhooks'.

Amy pushed the boat out in order to get the tests and treatment needed to enable her to carry a baby. She already had children and had also previously endured four miscarriages. At thirty-five she felt the urgent need to 'crack on' so she found someone to help her. However, Amy shared important insights into the monetary cost of fertility:

We had the resources to find information and find someone who could help us. I think we spent in the region of €10,000 between tests, medication, everything like that ... I had booked an appointment with somebody in London that I had found on the internet – they test for killer cells and all this kind of thing. But that was going to be another €10,000. I do think if you have the courage and the strength to keep going you will get there but you also need a lot of money to facilitate it … there is no assistance from the government here in terms of IVF. There is one charity that helps but you have a very slim chance of hitting it. The other choice is to keep going without the medication and without the advice; you either hope for the best or seek expert advice at a cost and hope for the best there too.

When Gretta lost her twins she would have loved another baby. She said wistfully: 'I have never felt our family was complete.' In his interview also, her husband Leo shared how he has been impacted since the loss:

It's like that invisible person and I think that's the way it will be … another person there that's looking over your shoulder … it eases with time but you don't forget.

In relation to miscarriage, Serena believed she might have felt differently if the losses had continued. Going on to have more children allowed her to look back philosophically. 'It is just one of those things that happens,' she said of her discovery via a scan at fourteen weeks that her baby was no longer viable.

Reflection

Let us take a moment to reflect on what we are learning about the aftermath of loss through miscarriage or stillbirth. There is no mistaking the depth of desire to have another baby. It was made abundantly clear that parents do not want to 'replace' the baby they have lost; rather, it is that 'urge', the deep-seated desire to have another baby, to hold a baby, to fill the void. Parents were strenuous in their conviction that another baby does not make up for earlier losses.

We are reminded that the 'rainbow' pregnancy can be full of worry and anxiety. Such pregnancies 'come with a price' and the emotional 'cost' is realised in an uneasy nine months. Amy spoke about how the monetary cost of tests and medicine to help create the bodily conditions within which a pregnancy might happen can be exorbitant.

Grieving the death of your baby while coping with a new pregnancy is a highly charged journey sometimes overrun with guilt (Why could my body not carry my baby?) and also fear and worry that the same thing will happen again. It is no longer taken for granted that all will be well. Mothers and fathers remain in a high state of alert each step of the way, aptly described by Catherine as 'on tenterhooks'.

We need to be mindful of those like Gretta, who, having lost her twins, was left feeling that her family was incomplete. Some of you may also resonate with the message from Serena, who in hindsight and with two further healthy pregnancies was able to reconcile her loss at fourteen weeks as 'one of those things that happens'.

Before we move on to the next chapter, let us consider for a moment Grace's important reminder about the impact of the loss:

People do need to understand how intense the grief is when a woman loses a child … and the impact of grief is so powerful … I don't know that people accept that the loss of a baby who is only maybe nine weeks in development in the womb is a valid thing to grieve about … there is a limitation on how long you are expected to grieve. And so that means that people grieve in secret nearly and still carry the pain …

Grace's words conclude this chapter with a clear message – that the pain of loss at whatever stage of pregnancy is something we must attend to so that it is not silenced as it was for her and for so many others in this research.

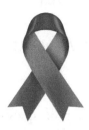

CHAPTER 5

'Why did my baby die?'

Why did it not go right? Was there something wrong?
Áine

You could feel the life stopping – it was awful …
Mary

There are many important questions that bereaved parents need answers to: Why did the miscarriage happen? Why did my baby die? Why did my baby die in the womb? Why did my baby die just hours before birth or during the birthing process or immediately afterwards? Post-mortems may not always provide the answers parents need as the cause of the loss may be indeterminable.

We can only imagine that those mums and dads who set their hearts on another baby would welcome feedback and therefore benefit from knowing what caused the miscarriage or stillbirth of their child. As we begin to explore the enlightening accounts, we learn that often the critical answers bereaved parents needed were difficult to come by. Knowing the cause of death remains an important part of the grieving process. Let us turn to some of the mums who shared their concerns.

'Why did it not go right?'

Bernadette and Beth wanted a clear reason why they lost their babies. Kathy lost four sons and no one really explained why. Bridget suffered fourteen miscarriages and an ectopic pregnancy before help was at hand.

Áine still gets angry that she had no feedback. She thought that having answers to her questions – Why did it not go right? Was there something wrong? – might help her 'rationalise' the miscarriage.

Ruth was expecting a boy when she miscarried at ten weeks. Regrettably, she was told: 'It happens to one in four; so don't worry, it's quite normal; you are lucky you had four already.'

Tara learned through her doctor that a combination of factors contributed to her miscarriages, including cysts on the ovaries and low progesterone levels. In an effort to understand what was going on, Tara read posts on the internet, but would advise that reading up is both 'helpful and unhelpful'. Any reassurance gained can be offset by other information that has the potential to create intense fear.

When she lost her baby in early pregnancy, Eimear concluded that 'it just wasn't meant to be'.

The need for answers

Bereaved mums and dads are sometimes haunted by questions such as: Why didn't we ask a second time? Why did we not push harder for answers? Apart from reliving the trauma through distress and flashbacks, sometimes having upsetting dreams and nightmares, feeling detached, emotionally numb or anxious, angry, guilty and upset, a key issue in any post-traumatic situation is this hypervigilance or being on high alert to make sure it does not happen again. This is a normal human response and it is very strong in the aftermath of loss. Indeed, at the heart of the trauma is loss because life will never be the same again.

This stands out in my mind as one of the key learnings from an enlightening six-week introduction to somatic experiencing (SE) with Bríd Keenan, an accredited somatic experiencing practitioner, based in Belfast. Bríd has a special interest in transgenerational trauma and many years' experience of working with traumatised clients. When a traumatic event pushes people past their normal capacity to cope, the shock state overwhelms them and the nervous system responds by going into 'freeze' mode. So the loss is held in the physiology of the body and takes its toll on mental, physical and emotional well-being. It is a state that is difficult to recover from and without healing can lead to longer-term health issues. It is reassuring to know, however, that with proper support through treatment, traumatic shock will begin to disappear over time.

Somatic experiencing is a body–mind therapeutic approach, developed by psychologist Peter Levine. SE focuses on healing trauma by helping the client/patient draw their attention to their body (where the trauma is held). The Hungarian-Canadian physician, expert on trauma and author Gabor Maté uses the analogy of the 'archaeology' of the traumatised mind that requires careful work – which he describes as gently dusting off tiny objects/fragments one by one – that, in the end, may restore it to a complete whole.

When parents agree to a post-mortem, it is an anxious time as they wait to hear the results. Anna waited eleven weeks to hear that there was 'no medical explanation' for the death of baby Gerry. He was induced at thirty-two weeks and born a healthy-sized 4 lb 4 oz baby. Similarly, Maura felt confused when she delivered Ronan, 'a perfect wee baby', at eighteen weeks. 'Did I do this?' she asked herself. It was a stressful time in her life.

Parents need answers so that they can take steps, as Drew said, to work towards prevention in the future and raise awareness too. Sometimes, the reason for the loss is hard to bear.

Drew and Jo struggled when they learned that the amniotic fluid, a protector and essential source of nutrients for the baby, had gradually 'gone' over the course of the pregnancy. This resulted in infection that had gathered around Zach's heart and brain. Drew recalled how Zach went through a night of 'wriggling' where he was probably struggling for breath, struggling for oxygen, as the fluid at that stage had completely gone. Concern about retention of fluids had been expressed by Drew and Jo to the midwife six weeks earlier; however, the conclusion was that Jo was 'low risk' and therefore no action was taken.

Shauna agreed to a post-mortem to know why Branna died at forty weeks and five days. When no cause was found, it made it harder for her to understand why it had happened, especially when Branna was a healthy weight and there was no cord around her neck.

An intrauterine growth restriction was the reason given to Betty and Tony to explain why baby Joshua died. At some point the placenta stopped working, stopped supporting his growth. He was 4 lbs 13 ozs when he was born. The medics reportedly ruled out genetic problems, blood problems and risk factors. To this day, the reason for the placenta not working remains a mystery.

'You know best, you are the mother'

The post-mortem on Leonie Ellen showed that Tess had strep B infection, a bacteria carried by the mother in the intestine and vagina. When Leonie Ellen was checked by the midwife, she was perfect; she had no physical abnormalities. The consultant explained that perhaps Tess's amniotic wall was not strong enough and that the infection may have got in through it. Strep B is not routinely tested for and Tess is adamant that it should be as it can pass in the birthing canal and cause the baby to die. She went on to say that strep B cannot be prevented but identification of it means that subsequent pregnancies can be treated through intravenous (IV) antibiotics which can be administered when the labour begins, to protect mother and baby. Tess delivered a strong, clear message:

Don't be fobbed off; know your body; keep persisting and always follow your own instincts. You know best, you are the mother. Always take care of yourself and your baby. If you have ever any doubts, keep going back … ask, be persistent.

It is important for mothers to trust their instincts, to seek information on all available tests and interventions they may require and to ensure that they receive what they need.

Clinical report upsetting

Leo and Gretta explained that baby Daniel, one of their twins, 'hadn't formed completely' but the other twin (Francis) was 'perfectly okay'. In Gretta's mind, she was twenty weeks into her pregnancy when Francis was born. However, the hospital report stated that Francis was consistent with a baby of sixteen weeks and that the baby was 'macerated' (meaning shrunken in). The 'clinical' language was upsetting and distressing. Leo decided not to read the report as it was 'not going to change anything'. Gretta however recommended that feedback be presented in a more sensitive way to bereaved parents. She shared a powerful insight into the internal, emotional tug of war that surrounds such documents:

> I really know I should shred it because it is something I never want my children to find after we are gone. But I can't bear to shred it because I feel that if I do, it's the end …

And in Gretta's poignant words, we see how tender a mother's heart is and how painful it is to let go or erase a connection with her baby, even if it is in the form of a report that is difficult to read.

When baby Sam was delivered at twenty-four weeks, Maria was concerned that scar tissue from a previous biopsy of cancerous cells had weakened her cervix. Regretfully, the medical team had not advised her to ensure that no pressure was put on her cervix while she was carrying baby Sam. Wistfully, she said: 'If only we had got to twenty-eight/twenty-nine weeks … but we will never know.'

'We pieced together the jigsaw'

In the aftermath of three miscarriages, the desperation to find out what was wrong – and hopefully provide solutions

– resulted in Catherine and Willie undertaking extensive research. Gradually they 'pieced together the jigsaw' of what was needed. The strong desire to have a second baby, to have a safe and successful pregnancy and deliver another baby safely into this world, was their driver. The investigation required extensive tests to be carried out, with all the attendant anxiety and stress that such testing can evoke, especially when it includes DNA and karyotype genetic testing.

Catherine and Willie learned that she had Robertsonian balanced translocation (a condition that one in 500 carry but may not be aware of), which means that when a pregnancy is coming together there is not enough genetic material for the foetus to continue to grow. The couple felt fortunate to have had a child already but realised that if any future pregnancies progressed, there was a strong possibility that the babies could be born with severe disabilities, and/or be incompatible with life. While there was relief in knowing more, it was difficult to take on board that there was a genetic disorder for which there was no cure.

Catherine persevered and took the recommended drugs to make her body fertile, including Utrogestan, Duphaston, Estrofem, Predison and Fraxiparine, as well as pre-pregnancy vitamins. She advised strongly however that there is a need to get mentally, emotionally and physically prepared, as it is a very difficult and unsettling process to endure. Letting go of her 'three wee babies' was part of her preparation. With the help of medical science, Willie and Catherine now have 'two more beautiful children', siblings to their first son.

Amy too wanted an explanation for her miscarriages and found that testing was the only way to find out what was going on. Visits to clinics in her locality had enabled her to become pregnant but each had ended in miscarriage. While her fourth pregnancy was more hopeful, at the twelve-week scan there was sadly no heartbeat. Deciding that 'enough was enough', Amy found a consultant in Dublin whose expertise is recurrent miscarriage. Two important outcomes emerged through testing: she learned that she had polycystic ovary syndrome (PCOS) that is due to a combination of genetic and environmental factors. In follow-up, intralipids were administered through a drip to help calm the immune system and nurture the body. A variety of medical interventions meant that Amy gave birth to 'a lovely little boy'. She and her husband were so delighted with the results they decided to try again. When her son was ten weeks old she re-started the same interventions and became pregnant again with her little girl. A happy ending for the family.

Of her own volition, Cecilia made the decision to seek out genetic testing. She learned that her previous loss was due to Turner syndrome (which affects only females and is characterised by one of the X chromosomes being missing or partially missing) and that it had a 1 per cent chance of happening again. Cecilia was angry when her doctor had questioned her choice to get tested – 'Who said you could do that?' She was firm in her rationale that she was not going to wait, and worked from the premise that you need to do things for yourself as no-one else is going to do them for you.

Bridget endured fourteen miscarriages and an ectopic pregnancy. In one of her last pregnancies, a referral by a junior doctor to a professor in Paddington Hospital, London proved to be insightful. The blood tests and scans revealed a condition known as antiphospholipid syndrome. That is, Bridget's blood was clotting, allowing her to get only so far in her pregnancies.

When she became pregnant, a clot formed in the placenta, causing it to 'break away', and as a result she lost her babies. The solution was injections of anticoagulants to keep the blood thin. The dosage is determined by height, build and other medical conditions.

Alarm bells going off

Mary's baby Emmet Pio was not swallowing the amniotic fluid. As a result, Mary was 'humungous', to the point that it was impacting upon her ability to breathe easily. Emmet Pio had arthrogryposis syndrome, meaning crooked limbs; it is a form of Edwards syndrome is known as Trisomy 18. Foetal akinesia deformation sequence (FADS) was also mentioned. This is a condition characterised by a decrease in foetal movement and intrauterine growth restriction as well as joint contractions, underdevelopment of the lungs and other developmental factors. At twenty-five weeks, Mary's waters broke and she was 'blue lighted' to the hospital seventy miles away. In the midst of it all, she could feel baby Emmet Pio letting go of life: 'I could feel his wee limbs stopping ... you could feel the life stopping ...'

Another couple who found themselves confronted with the difficulties arising from Edwards syndrome were John and Emily. Around twenty-three weeks into the pregnancy, they learned that baby Caoimhe's chromosome disorder was associated with this condition. Caoimhe would not survive outside the womb, or at least not for long anyway. John and Emily knew from previous discussions with the consultant that Caoimhe's heart was on her right-hand side (known as dextrocardia) and that she had a hole in her heart – shocking and upsetting news at the time. Although John and Emily were initially optimistic that the prognosis with this heart condition was for a 'normal life', at a later stage when the nurse phoned with the results and said 'I'm really sorry to say but your baby has Edwards syndrome. Do you know what it means?', Emily screamed as she knew her baby was going to die.

Lilly believed that the death of her baby girl, Amilia Rose, born 1 lb weight at twenty-eight weeks, was due to neglect. She learned that the placenta had clotted with blood and her baby was consequently starved, and she believes the concerns she expressed about her baby could have been taken more seriously. It was particularly difficult to discover that an earlier scan had revealed that Amilia was small, and Lilly believes an attempt should have been made to save her at that stage.

In Rose's case, an impact review had to be carried out, such were the complexities of the case of Ellen born at thirty-eight weeks. Some important lessons were learned as a result and implemented into regulations at the hospital. Concerned that she wasn't detecting any movement from her baby, Rose came to the hospital and was scanned in A&E; however, she was advised that she would have to wait four hours for follow-up. Feeling anxious about leaving her children for a lengthy period with her mum, Rose decided not to wait. She left the hospital at seven o'clock and learned later that 'not there' was recorded in her file when she was called three and a half hours later at ten-thirty. In bed that night she felt Ellen move.

Reflection

When we suffer a traumatic event we need to understand what happened and why it happened, to enable us to process it fully and make sense of the tragedy. Bereaved parents *need to know* why their baby died. This might explain why many agree to a post-mortem even though that decision is not an easy one. The thought of their tiny baby being exposed to an autopsy is unbearable. However, desperate for answers, some will make the choice and sign the permission paper.

Sometimes the medical profession may suggest a post-mortem so that they too can learn about the possible cause of death. However, it is vexing when the results – often long-awaited – do not reveal the answers that are longed for; or sometimes results are not reported back at all. In either case, parents remain in a kind of information limbo and feel let down. How might we feel if we were waiting on significant and important results that were not forthcoming?

We know that on the journey through pregnancy, parents rely on medical guidance and trust the expert knowledge of the health professionals. Let us also remember that it creates profound unease and deep concern when bereaved mothers and fathers come to the conclusion that decisions made by the health professionals during the pregnancy could have contributed to the death of their baby.

It is unacceptable for a miscarriage to be dismissed with a statistic such as 'it happens to one in four'; or that the decision to undergo genetic testing is subjected to a pertinent question from a medic: 'Who said you could do that?' Surely it is the right of the mother and father to make that choice. Why is the approval of the health professional necessary when time is of the essence and there is a desire to 'crack on' and get testing started? Indeed we could speculate: if the medic *was* consulted in the first instance, what might the response have been? Positive or negative? Supportive or unsupportive?

Regardless of the psychological or monetary cost, parents will strenuously engage with testing to ensure that they create the optimal health conditions within which a pregnancy becomes possible. The detailed accounts of the testing undertaken and follow-up medications demonstrate the determination to understand what makes their body tick and to illuminate the medical mysteries that prevent a healthy pregnancy.

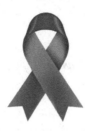

CHAPTER 6

'The silence was deafening'

*Even though I knew she was dead I still expected her to cry
or to move ...*
Lilly

There wasn't a peep ...
Mary

When we hear of an expected baby having a fatal foetal condition our thoughts turn immediately to the parents. We know that such conditions affect the health and well-being of the baby and can cause death or result in a form of disease after the birth. We may not fully understand the nature of the baby's illness as there are a multitude of fatal foetal conditions. However, the news makes us sad for those who have to live with the knowledge that their baby's survival is unlikely that their baby is unwell and most likely will not be born alive. We might feel intensely emotional as we attempt to put ourselves in the shoes of these grieving parents. Indeed, our immediate reaction might be to dismiss the disturbing thoughts and 'escape' as quickly as possible. We know there are parents in this book and readers too who cannot escape, as they have lived the experience and *know* what it is like to go through the trauma of stillbirth. There is a desire among those who *do know* that others would be understanding, empathic and sensitive to the meaning of loss.

Before we continue, let us take a moment to consider these questions:

- Can any of us even begin to imagine how *we* might cope if we were on a similar journey? If we knew that our precious baby was not going to live?

- Can *we*, for a moment, put ourselves in the shoes of the mums and dads who go through the pregnancy knowing that their baby will be birthed in silence without life or breath?

- Can *we* comprehend the enormity of what it means to give birth to a son or daughter who will not be alive when they arrive in this world, or who might draw their last breath moments after being birthed?

These are very difficult questions that have the capacity to shift us into uneasy territory. In this chapter, mothers and fathers speak of the unnerving – even frightening – journey in the lead-up to the birth and the birth itself. For some it was a confusing time, unsure what to expect yet knowing that the outcome was going to be sad and emotional. As Mary reminds us, it is 'traumatic' knowing that you are going to give birth but knowing too that your baby is not going to live.

Before we come to the 'voices' of the parents, it seems timely here to draw on Seamus Heaney's lament 'Elegy for a Still-Born Child', in which the poet helps us to enter the world of bereaved parents through a different route, as it were. Poetry has the power to shake us up, to stop us in our tracks, to drive home a message that enters our emotional world, sometimes like a bolt out of the blue. Heaney addresses the stillborn child as he movingly illustrates the physical, mental and emotional 'cost' for both mother and father, and in doing so illuminates the painful journey beyond the loss of a baby.

The lament begins:

Your mother walks light as an empty creel
Unlearning the intimate nudge and pull

Your trussed-up weight of seed-flesh and bone-curd
Had insisted on. That evicted world
Contracts round its history, its scar.

The expectant mother is intimately connected to her growing baby's presence in her body. Every move, kick and stretch reassures her and brings acute awareness of the blossoming new life. The 'intimate nudge and pull' is encoded in a mother's mind long after the painful ending. Unlearning will not be easily achieved as the child remains 'present' in its devastating absence. Steeped in grief at the empty chasm of her womb, 'that evicted world' continues to remind the mother of her loss. In eight paradoxical words, the poet signals the mental and emotional weight:

Your mother heavy with the lightness in her.

Two couplets make up the second section of the poem and Heaney once again addresses the child to convey how his friend, the father-in-waiting, is profoundly impacted:

For six months you stayed cartographer
Charting my friend from husband towards father.

He guessed a globe behind your steady mound.
Then the pole fell, shooting star, into the ground.

With each month of pregnancy, the child is the 'cartographer' mapping out, as it were, a new future role for his father to cherish and be proud of; no longer a husband only, but a father in the making. The poet reflects on the hopeful father who, in observing the 'steady mound' of the child growing within his mother's womb, feels the attachment to the child that allows him to imagine the vast potential and possibilities that the new baby would bring.

In the final section, we learn of the poet's own reflections on the loss (where he speaks directly to the reader):

On lonely journeys I think of it all
Birth of death, exhumation for burial;

Who could not fail to be moved by such heart-touching lines, through which Heaney expresses the tragic reality of loss that bereaved parents endure. Stillbirth, the 'birth of death'. A birth is normally associated with joy and celebration, but when you know your child is to be born without life or breath, when your child is to be 'exhumed', brought forth from the womb to be buried, the grief is unspeakable.

In the course of the interviews, I was deeply touched to hear mothers and fathers speak of the 'perfect' little babies that they gave birth to. To deliver a beautiful baby but be denied the opportunity to know that little being must be unbearable. Mothers spoke about how the joy and happiness normally associated with the arrival of a newborn was agonisingly absent. The two quotes at the top of the chapter bring home to us how excruciatingly painful a time this is for parents. The stories are profoundly touching and will no doubt be read with empathy and compassion. Please take care of yourself as you continue reading this chapter.

'It's like a car crash'

When John and Emily knew that their little girl Caoimhe was not going to live, John likened the journey through pregnancy towards birth to a car crash:

> The car is going and we know it is going and we just don't know when it is going to crash but we know it is not going to end well … we both know … devastating.

John went on to describe the sensation of standing alone in the hospital and the world whirling around him:

> When you are the parent standing in the hospital and fifty-five or sixty people are running past you at different times doing different jobs and completely ignoring you, it's very like that montage in a film where the person is alone, standing there, cameras sped up all around and everyone is just going by. What the hell is going on here? Just say something rather than say nothing! I think that's really, really important.

Anna was sent home and told to come back when she was ready for her baby to be delivered. She felt for her husband Paul, aware that it was 'every bit as bad if not worse for him' waiting and watching as baby Gerry arrived 'perfectly formed, 4 lb 4 ozs and lovely'. The opportunity to spend as much time as they wanted with Gerry was important, welcomed and appreciated in the hours after the birth. Babies are born to be held in their parents' arms, to be examined, pressed against the heart, spoken to and have their spirits reassured that they are as cherished, loved and wanted as any child. The grieving process for parents who have the opportunity to spend time with their baby is normalised and eased by this moment of togetherness.

'You don't want to let go … and you have to let go'

Maria knew that baby Sam would not have a chance at life. When he was born the only sound in the room was Maria's. In that moment, she knew that she would have to let him go:

> The actual second of his birth I just remember the sound was guttural … the noise I made – once he was born he was gone, because I couldn't keep him anymore – that was it, it was over. Physically, that second, my heart just broke.

Cecilia's baby Alex was born 'fully formed' at twenty-three weeks and weighed 1 lb 10 ozs. Cecelia described the 'horrific experience' of going in and not having the child crying in the room. She felt that people need a 'heads up' about stillbirth. Her immediate feeling was one of anger and frustration, knowing that once her baby was born she had to let her go:

> Everything just goes straight through you; frustration … floods of tears … all emotions are there but mainly anger because they are taking her away from you. Anger because you don't want to let go … and you have to let go.

Mary and Liam knew that baby Emmet Pio's lungs had not developed properly and he would not survive. When he was born Mary remembered how 'the silence was deafening':

There wasn't a peep … a midwife in the corner was breaking her heart … I didn't know whether to cry or … And I couldn't get up. There was another midwife by my side … the doctor … and all these machines.

Having agreed to take gas and air for the first time, along with an epidural, Rose was unprepared for the reaction she experienced:

I remember looking down on myself in the delivery room, it was as if I was floating on the ceiling and thinking to myself, *Oh my God, am I dying here too?* Is there something happening to me that I am not kind of realising? It was like I was in a dream … going through the motions … crying on and off …

Rose had an out-of-body experience during the birthing process. Such experiences can be trauma-related and seen as a coping mechanism when trauma is present. This *was* a traumatic situation – Rose knew that her baby had died and would be born without life.

As soon as Ellen was born she was dressed and taken away for a post-mortem. When Rose later heard other mums at Féileacáin (Stillbirth and Neonatal Death Association of Ireland) speak about bathing their babies, she regrets not having had more time with her daughter after the birth. If the opportunity is taken away from parents to bond with the spirit of their baby, there is no second chance. It makes it even more difficult to find out later that they might have had more time. It also adds unnecessary guilt, as if they should have known, should have asked and should have demanded that right. This makes it so important that hospital policy recognises the rights of parents to make their own decisions after such births and that they not be hurried in such decision-making.

'Be prepared for the silence in the room'

Emily's midwife provided her with the kind of support that Cecilia and Maria craved. The midwife had advised Emily to 'be prepared for the silence in the room after your baby is born'. There was 'pure silence' when Caoimhe arrived, as she died during the final stage of the delivery. With this realisation, Emily said to her husband, 'John, we are not going to hear her cry.' Emily recalled:

> The feeling in my body was surreal ... it was literally like I felt her life leave me, I just felt an emptiness ... I knew because she had been kicking, she had been moving and I knew ... Bear in mind there were no machines; they said it would be too distracting to have machines in the room whereby you would have heard her in distress.

During her labour with Joshua, the caring and compassionate staff were as helpful as they could be, Betty recalled. The midwives helped release the pressure and tension with humour. However, prior to going into the ward, Betty found it hard to be in a waiting area with other mums who were going in to deliver a healthy baby, a situation that was very unwelcome at the time.

Bernadette too shared a 'very clear memory' of being in the labour ward and hearing other mothers screaming in pain. She reflected:

After the final big push there was always the beautiful sound of a baby crying. When I gave birth to baby Aoife the only sound was me crying ... I will never forget it.

This begs the question about separate delivery facilities for these mothers and fathers. It takes so little to protect parents from the starkness of being with a silent baby in a delivery room while around them the cries of newborns are heard.

Why, parents may well ask, is this not available in every hospital in all of Ireland? Why, when it would help, could it not be done? Thankfully, some hospitals have started to introduce 'bereavement suites' in the maternity wings. These compact suites comprise a bedroom, kitchen and bathroom – a comprehensive facility separated from the main maternity ward that ensures privacy during a deeply sensitive time.

'I wanted to feel labour pain'

When Lilly was told she could be given 'loads of meds and drugs' to induce labour because her baby was not alive, she reacted firmly: 'I don't want any drugs.' When Amilia arrived it was an emotional tug of war between wishful thinking and reality:

I wanted to feel labour pain ... and my labour was very slow ... It was such a sin to see her there lifeless. Even though I knew she was dead I still expected her to cry or to move.

On the way home from the hospital, Lilly nursed baby Amilia's coffin. Partly, she was too scared to hold her daughter in case she hurt her or her baby 'fell apart'. However, Lilly wishes now she had asked the nurse to lift Amilia out so that she could have held her in her arms. So many of these decisions could be made in advance if we listened to mothers prior to and at the time of birth, and to their feedback afterwards.

Reflection

This chapter reflects on one of the most traumatic times for any parent: delivering a beloved baby, born without life; saying goodbye and 'letting go'. It has to be remembered that the loss of a baby at whatever stage in the pregnancy leaves a psychological scar, an indelible mark that cannot be erased. In a collaborative study with the University of Southern Denmark and the National Center for Psychotraumatology in Denmark, Siobhan Murphy and Mark Shevlin of Ulster University studied a sample of 455 parents bereaved of a baby. The study showed that for up to five years after the loss of a baby, bereaved parents suffer with symptoms of depression, anxiety, dissociation, sleep disturbances, somatisation – and in particular interpersonal sensitivity and aggression.

The challenging questions posed at the outset of this chapter are important – they are intended to stir the mind and encourage us to think ahead of the stories we are about to read. We turned to Seamus Heaney's elegy in which the poet addressed the unborn child to help us gain perspective on the traumatic impact of loss on parents.

Let us pause now and 'hear' these poignant reflections from Betty and Maria …

Walking out with empty arms … people would have just thought you were there for an appointment … but we knew that we were missing our baby and since then it's exactly what it felt like – there's just a hole.

Betty

Round about Christmas I was really struggling within my-self. I found Archie's grief on top of my grief so hard to handle. I just couldn't cope with his and mine. I just needed something for myself. So I rang Cruse Bereavement Care.

Maria

Maria's recognition that she needed help by phoning Cruse Bereavement Care shows how crucial it is that people have support to help them cope with such an enormous loss.

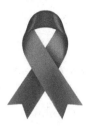

CHAPTER 7

'Say my baby's name'

You just want your baby's life to be recognised as human, as real, as worthwhile. And that they weren't any less a person.

Sarrah

We always should say the baby's name because that's what we want to hear. It's our child after all ...

John

We often hear the expression, what's in a name? The short answer is – everything! As we know, our name represents our identity and individuality; it is a statement of who we are and where we came from. Our first and last names confirm our lineage, our heritage. When our name is known and remembered, it is the ultimate form of recognition and acknowledgement.

We know that the choice of a name for an expected baby is one of the most important decisions parents will make. There could be a favourite baby name that has been harboured for a long time. Sometimes we hear declarations such as: 'If ever I have a boy, I'm going to call him —; if ever I have a girl, I'm going to call her —.' Whatever way the decision is arrived at, the name of that much-wanted baby is significant.

When an adult dies, we often commiserate with their loved ones and speak openly about the deceased. No wonder parents ask why it is taboo to speak about a baby who is lost through miscarriage or stillbirth. It is also the loss of a cherished human life – a loss that bereaved parents live with every day. Parents are not unwell or sick, they are grieving, so to avoid them or to avoid mentioning their baby is deeply wounding. Parents crave recognition and validation of their lost child. They long to hear their baby's name.

We need to remember that people who are mourning a baby do not 'get over' the loss. In the literature, I came across the expression 'invisible earthquake' to describe what happens internally when parents lose a baby. It struck me as a powerful analogy that quantifies and qualifies the emotional, mental and physical trauma of stillbirth and miscarriage. The trauma remains unseen by other people. It is only fully known to the mum or dad and perhaps somewhat visible within the close family network.

There are many myths about grief – about its nature, its intensity, its duration, its stages. It is known that there is not a predictable or linear journey through what is recognised as the stages of grief. As many have reported over the years, it is almost as if those affected go through shock, denial, the what-ifs, anger and depression all in the space of an hour, or over the course of a day. This hourly or daily 'cycle' may occur and re-occur for a long time before any sense of peace or acceptance appears on the horizon. The inability of family or friends to deal with the pain of the bereaved can add an extra dimension to their suffering. People need to know that it is a terrible feeling when that much-wanted baby is discounted. It is painful, Sarrah said, when 'nobody wants to listen, nobody cares, [the baby is] not seen, not there, not human, not worth it really'. Everyone means well but it is important to know that speaking about a baby who has died will not hurt parents – it is *not* speaking about the baby, as we are about to find out, that can cause the most pain.

Please don't 'skirt around' the loss

Maria found it annoying that people would sometimes cross the street to avoid her; or if they *did* talk they would 'skirt around' the loss. She was firm in her mind that she was not going to deny her child 'because someone else is feeling uncomfortable'. Parents do not want people to avoid them or keep a distance, and they readily dismiss the perception that it might cause hurt or offence to mention the baby. Hearing the baby's name is an important part of the grieving process as the child remains part of the family, forever. He or she is remembered, celebrated and spoken about, as Bridget reminds us, on a daily basis, including at birthdays, anniversaries and at Christmas.

Here we find out more from those who know best – those who have been bereaved – about the importance of recognising and validating lost babies.

Drew succinctly stated his plea, that echoes the wishes of many bereaved parents: 'Say my baby's name.' He went on:

We love to hear him called by his name; we love to hear people saying 'Zach'.

Sarrah explained the need that exists within every bereaved parent:

Your heart is aching and breaking ... you just want your baby's life to be recognised as human, as real, as worthwhile. And that they weren't any less a person.

In addition, Sarrah warmly noted the example set by Sands:

In meeting and supporting parents, Sands always acknowledge and refer to the baby by name.

It has to be remembered that it is not always easy for bereaved parents to bring up their baby's name in the course of conversation. It may be on a day or at a time when feelings of grief and loss are at the surface. On these days, parents may be reluctant to talk. People around the bereaved may attempt to cope with their personal discomfort by talking about their own losses! What is needed is sensitivity, awareness and a listening ear. Saying something such as 'I am sorry your baby [name] died' is a very acceptable, sympathetic response. Or if the name of the baby is unknown, parents would like to be asked: 'What did you call him?' 'What did you call her?'

What angers Tess is the attitude of those who think that naming babies is futile, especially when the gender of the child is unknown.

> People think we are crazy but I don't care. It has never happened to them and, in my mind, I think, well, when you have put three of them in the ground then you can judge me.

That said, Tess understands how difficult it can be for people to talk about death and loss. However, being censored in relation to speaking of her baby elicited a strong response:

> When anybody dies, people don't know what to say, whether it's a baby, an older person, or a middle-aged person. Death is one of those subjects; I think it depends on your own upbringing, how you have been brought up, whether you are able to talk about death or not. My father passed away twelve years ago and if I talk about him that's perfectly fine. But if I talk about my daughter in some respects I

am perceived as weird. Why are you talking about a dead baby? I have had good experiences where people have said nice things. I have really only had one very bad experience where someone told me not to talk about it. It just pushed a button and made me flip.

Parents make a personal decision on whether or not to name their child. For those who took part in this study, naming often depended on the duration of the pregnancy and whether or not the baby's gender was known. Some felt that naming the baby and assigning a gender was very helpful. In some cases of very early loss, mums went with their 'gut' and speculated on whether they were expecting a boy or a girl and named the baby accordingly.

The importance of naming was particularly acute in Bridget's case. She is incredibly proud of all fifteen children that she conceived and lost; she felt it necessary in the end to give each an identity by name:

I have named all fifteen of them now. I didn't at the start but then because I had Conor and Charlie and they had names, I thought all my babies needed names. So they all begin with C – I don't know why. Whenever I go up to Conor and Charlie's graves I put fifteen roses in each of their plots. On World Miscarriage Day I put fifteen wee angels on my posts, or fifteen kisses – it marks them all.

John, who wants to send out positive messages, suggests that perhaps parents should pave the way by being comfortable themselves in saying their baby's name, and in speaking about and 'celebrating' their child:

We always should say the baby's name because that's what we want to hear. It's our child, after all … people would say 'your baby died', but no one ever says Caoimhe. Always celebrate your child and always talk about things, don't bottle things up.

Reflection

Bereaved parents are asking for a gesture that would mean the world to them, that is, to hear people say their baby's name, acknowledge the existence of their baby. We need to respect their wishes for validation of the baby that did not survive, a new life that was waiting to be welcomed into their world. Anyone who has been bereaved can recount the ways in which people avoided them or the extraordinary things that were said to them by people who genuinely cared for them and wanted to console them. In the wish to say something positive, some might offer unspeakably inappropriate comments such as 'Sure, you are young, you'll have another.'

We know that very often people feel awkward and self-conscious when meeting the bereaved. People mean well – but often they are stuck and unsure, afraid to offend or hurt. What really hurts the bereaved is avoidance, when people cross to the other side of the street, not mentioning the baby at all or, as Maria said, 'skirting around' the loss in conversation. The bereaved are pleading for people to engage and to mention the baby's name, if it is known.

We also need to note John's wise words that bereaved parents themselves could help reduce the stress and awkwardness through leading by example – talking about their baby, mentioning the baby's name, not bottling things up.

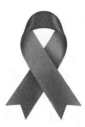

CHAPTER 8

Bereaved Siblings: 'You live for the living'

It is known that the loss of a baby through stillbirth or miscarriage impacts on family members and the wider family network. We know that each child, like each adult, is a unique individual and may understand death and loss in keeping with their own life experiences. A child who has lost a beloved pet may know the feelings that come with an ending, including shock, sadness, anger, guilt or fear. That said, a child's ability to put their feelings into words may vary according to their age and stage of development. It is recognised that, as with adults, children respond to loss in a unique and personal way. We know that just as parents have a 'huge need' to speak about the baby, the same need exists in many children.

Insights from studies in bereavement, loss and grief teach us that the very young are deeply affected when a significant person in their life 'disappears'. Loss can impact on a child's short-term and longer-term psychological health and well-being, including levels of anxiety, self-esteem and acting-out behaviour. As the deeply touching accounts in this chapter will show, when the excitement of the prospect of a new baby brother or sister turns into sadness, it takes a toll on children. Bernadette's example tenderly illustrates this point.

While Bernadette's older children fully embrace that they have a baby sister 'in heaven', there has been 'heartache' along the way. Bernadette's eldest child struggled emotionally after his baby sister Aoife was born at twenty-two weeks. When Bernadette subsequently became pregnant with a little baby girl her son became very protective, and sensitive to his mum's form and moods: 'It was a lot of worry on a young boy's shoulders.' The birth of his sister, however, brought healing as it helped him, his siblings and all the family to witness pregnancy as 'a happy time and a beautiful person brought into the world from it'.

Research shows that when a sibling dies, children will experience a wide range of feelings including anger, grief and frustration. Some may feel vulnerable and in turn suffer with 'survivor guilt' that may be expressed in questions: Why my brother and not me? Why my sister and not me? Another difficulty for surviving children is that their parents may 'retreat' into their own grief, rendering them 'unavailable' to the child. Rose recalled the wise counsel offered by a consultant in relation to her bereaved children:

> The boys should always feel that she [the baby] is there to talk to and ... if they feel like sitting at the grave ... and having a chat and want to talk to her or feel like talking about her at home – that's good for them.

The loss of a baby creates an ongoing internal anxiety in parents about the health and well-being of the living children that in turn shapes future relationships. As Bernadette discovered, the experience of loss and the emotional impact that ensues affects the entire family in an 'underlying way'. She became 'massively over-protective' and was only comfortable leaving her children with her mother or childminder.

As we engage with the stories we learn how siblings ensured that their brother or sister was not forgotten. The baby was spoken about daily, prayed for, remembered on birthdays and anniversaries, their grave visited regularly.

One of the key behavioural learning concepts in psychology is role-modelling and how babies and children model the behaviour of the adults around them. The tender image of the toddler who learned to imitate and emulate her pregnant mum touched me deeply.

'I am like Mammy, I have a baby'

When children understand that there is another baby coming into the family, they are excited at the prospect. Shauna explained that she had prepared her little girl so much for the arrival of her new sister, that one day she found her walking around with a pillow up her jumper saying: 'I am like Mammy, I have a baby.'

When her daughter learned that the baby had gone to 'live with God in heaven', she did not ask any questions. Neither did she speak about the baby when she was brought home to be waked. It can be hard for a two-year-old to articulate what they are feeling inside but we could speculate that her silence indicated sadness or grief. As she got older she opened up more; she even tried to explain things to her younger brother when they visited the baby's grave. He appeared to be less inquisitive and 'quite laid back', leading Shauna to conclude that maybe 'wee boys are different'. In later years, when her daughter asked to see photographs of her sister she became upset. Shauna explained her rationale for sharing pictures with her daughter:

She didn't know why her sister died; she didn't know what she was like ... maybe she was thinking was she deformed? So, to see a perfectly normal wee baby set her mind at rest.

Sharing a photo when a sibling requests it or offering a reasonable explanation about the baby could end years of worry and anxiety that a child may have been harbouring. Shauna was clear that she would at some point in the future also tell her youngest daughter about her sister.

Like Shauna, Cecilia believed in being open about baby Alex. In her view, it is better to explain to children sooner rather than later: 'If you leave it too long, it gets harder to say.' Cecilia did not want her children to be afraid to come to her and ask about their sister. When the question 'Who's in there?' arose on family visits to the grave, the siblings were told about their sister. Cecilia credits her son, who was a toddler at the time of the death, with 'getting her through' as without him she does not know how she might have ended up. It was his plea, 'Mummy, you need to be up', and his encouragement of her to get out of bed in the morning that gave 'purpose' to her day.

Serena too had her own reasons for 'not hiding the loss' from her children: 'I think it is better to be out there.' Serena found that when she spoke openly about the post-natal depression she suffered after her first child, it helped others to open up. Serena applied the same philosophy to speaking about her miscarriage. Opening up in this way releases the emotions and in turn helps other people, who may never have spoken up before, to express their feelings.

The value of speaking up honestly and age-appropriately with children is reinforced throughout the research. Grace made sure that her daughter was comforted by knowing that as Daniel's twin they would probably have looked alike and that she also had a big sister, Caoimhe.

Rose learned how important it is to be sensitive to how siblings respond to the death of a baby. In the hospital her boys would not go near their sister, perhaps unsure how to react or respond. However, when baby Ellen was brought home they reacted differently – they asked questions and wanted to know more about her.

Inquisitiveness in children about the baby needs to be respected and responded to as honestly as possible in an age-appropriate way. The questions children ask may trigger sadness in a parent. Nevertheless, responding helps children to understand the loss, and as they grow older they will appreciate having been included rather than excluded.

However, raising the topic of loss and communicating with children is especially difficult when parents are struggling with their own emotions, as Maura found out. Her daughters knew there was a baby coming. Maura then had to tell them about the loss:

I was traumatised, in an awful state … I had to tell them and they were heartbroken.

When to initiate conversation

Ruth found it impossible to talk. As a mum, she is supportive and understanding and wants the best for her children. However, she carries hidden angst and guilt that she 'lost their sibling'; she feels responsible for the loss and therefore after such a long time finds it too difficult to bring up the conversation.

Ruth is not alone in her struggle. Beth, aware of her children's emotionality, initially declined to say anything. It took her a long time to tell her children and with the passage of time it became more difficult. Eventually she found the strength, not just to tell them, but also to write about the loss of her baby.

Eimear was glad not to have to tell her children when she miscarried on New Year's Eve. At the time, her children were playing with their Christmas toys downstairs and were oblivious to what was going on. She was thankful that they did not know and that no explanation was needed. Later, when she did tell them, her daughter responded sympathetically as she was already aware of someone who had suffered a miscarriage. Young as she was at the time, Eimear's daughter was 'quite grown up for her age' and was able to reflect and commiserate with her mum, especially when first communion time came around. Eimear valued that support.

Anna explained that baby Gerry's little brother was so anxious to talk about him *all the time* at school, the teacher had to confine speaking about Gerry to morning prayers.

He would be quite fascinated talking about Gerry ... Gerry should have been older and able to play football. All the wee ones at night pray – 'God bless Mammy and Daddy'.

It is not unusual for families to name all the children in birth order at night prayers and this means that a baby that is lost is kept in the family in a special way.

'They sense ... that you still hurt'

In anticipation of their brother's arrival, Mary's children kept toys, Matchbox cars and hurling sticks for him. At the sad news of Emmet Pio's death, the siblings were 'broken-hearted'. When it came to closing the lid of the coffin, the siblings touchingly put in a Matchbox car, a rainbow loom band made by one of his brothers, and his sister's All-Ireland medal that she won for playing football. Mary noted that since the loss, her two young sons are like 'sticking plasters'. When she sits down to relax at night they sit on either side of her on the sofa, a gesture she sees as her boys protecting and supporting her. 'They sense ... that you still hurt.' Children are not only concerned about the loss of their sibling, they also worry about the visible impact of the loss on their parents. While managing their own grief, children are sensitive to and want to support and care for their grieving parents. Significant questions can emerge from young, enquiring minds.

'Why is there a birthday cake when he is not here?'

Hearing their daughters talk about their brother Joshua is a source of comfort for Betty and Tony. At the annual celebration of Joshua's birthday where he was remembered and honoured with a picnic, ice-cream and a birthday cake, the question arose: 'Why is there a birthday cake when he is not here?' As their two daughters, who were young when Joshua was born, have got older, Betty and Tony realise that their innocent questions (and the explanations offered in return) have helped their daughters to 'work it all out' in their heads. Betty reflected on one of the girls studying a picture of her brother Joshua. As they all looked alike as babies, Betty was convinced that her daughter thought it was a picture of her!

'You live for the living'

Leo and Gretta's children too had a natural curiosity about the lost siblings. Before the loss, they 'debated' whether they would like a new brother or sister! Leo's thought was that attending to your children 'keeps you from being too absorbed in what you have lost … you never forget it, but you live for the living'. Keeping going for the sake of the children was also good, in Gretta's view, as being busy 'does really keep you pedalling'.

'Thank you for giving my mammy back to me'

Sands – the stillbirth and neonatal death service in Northern Ireland – gave Sarrah the courage she needed to start the process of telling her children about Grace. She recalled how her daughter was so appreciative of her mum opening up that she rang the organisation and thanked them for not only giving her mum the courage to speak but also for giving her mammy 'back' to her. Telling her adult sons, on the other hand, was a different matter for Sarrah. She did so with trepidation. One son responded with shock, then empathy; another with sympathy; there was a matter-of-fact response; and then with another son tears and hugs.

'Seventeen weeks'

During the pregnancy with their baby Caoimhe, John and Emily were told the traumatic news of Caoimhe's prognosis. John felt 'very lucky' to have seventeen weeks in which to digest the news but he is not sure which is the more 'heartbreaking' scenario: going into hospital expecting to come out three days later with a newborn baby and that not happening, or having seventeen weeks to adjust to the news that your baby is not going to live.

Both he and Emily were determined, not only to help their girls, aged eight and five at the time, through the trauma, but to 'include' them as much as possible in the lead-up to the birth and beyond. This approach had 'the best possible outcome' as Caoimhe continues to be part of the family, she is spoken about daily and will never be forgotten. Their story is shared here as readers may find the insights helpful.

Caoimhe's story

Beginning the explanation in an appropriate way was a significant task as John and Emily knew that the news was going to turn their children's world upside-down as they had been telling everyone about the expected baby.

On the day the news was to be shared, Emily's sister had helped the children pick out two new teddies. Both Emily and John were physically sick as the moment approached. But slowly and carefully they told their children about the baby's condition. It was important to reassure them that their lives were not in danger or that the same thing was not going to happen to them. A multitude of feelings and a 'million questions' came up, including: 'Is the baby going to die? How can God do this?' Emily found a way to respond:

The baby could die … this is the Caoimhe we are being given. We have to love her the same way as we love each other. She will teach us to do it in a different way – I am sure along the way we will figure out the different lessons she is going to teach us.

John and Emily admitted they were 'winging it' as 'no one gives you a book'. Thinking ahead to the birth and not knowing if Caoimhe might still be alive, some very difficult questions emerged: What do we do if she is alive? Do we bring our daughters in? What if she dies in front of them?

'I know she is dead but isn't she lovely?'

When their new sister arrived home from the hospital in her Moses basket, Emily recalled how one of their daughters announced so poignantly:

Mam, I know she is dead but isn't she lovely?

To their parents' amazement, upset as they were, their children were 'straight in', kissing and cuddling their new sister. The next question asked was: 'What happens now?' John and Emily attended to their children's request to allow others to come and meet their new sister. However, it was important that they understood that some mourners might want to see Caoimhe and some might not; some people might be crying but later on they could be talking, smiling or laughing. To accommodate their children's desire to be close to their sister, on the night before the funeral they slept beside her on mattresses in their parents' bedroom; the following morning they had breakfast in the sitting room with their sister beside them.

On Caoimhe's birthday, the family have a day out doing 'something that the kids want to do'. Ensuring that Caoimhe remains part of the family is evident in all correspondence.

When their children phone their cousins and other relations to sing 'Happy Birthday', they say happy birthday from Caoimhe as well. Every card that is written has her name included at the bottom of the page with kisses and hugs. Emily concluded: 'We couldn't have hoped for any better than that. It's fantastic.' Everything associated with Caoimhe is important: the grave is her garden; her special song is Celine Dion's 'A Mother's Prayer'. Especially important are the teddies that say 'BIG SIS'. Emily found a way to reassure and comfort her daughters:

> When you are feeling scared, sad or feeling upset over something, you always know that Caoimhe is right there with you … for the rest of your life you are never alone.

Reflection

Children are:

- profoundly impacted by the news of a new sibling on the way;
- deeply affected when they learn about the loss;
- sensitive to parents following the loss of a baby;
- filled with emotions, questions and feelings that may remain unexpressed.

Children need:

- recognition that the trauma of the loss takes a psychological toll on them;

- to be told about the loss sooner rather than later; if it is left too long it is harder to say and it may never get said;

- their questions to be responded to sensitively (in keeping with their age or stage of development);

- to be included as much as possible, not excluded.

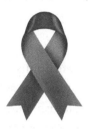

CHAPTER 9

Honouring My Child

It's about having something tangible, somewhere to go,
some way of remembering …

Grace

There are events and transitions in our lives – both happy and sad – that may stand out as huge landmarks. There are memories we cherish and others we recall with sadness. In this study the importance of creating memories was voiced very powerfully during the interviews. No matter how much or how little time they had in this world, lost babies 'remain forever' in the hearts and minds of parents who want to ensure that their baby is forever remembered. As Leo said:

They existed; they had their place here, albeit short; they had their presence …

As they navigate their way through the weeks and months beyond the loss, bereaved families choose different ways to remember and honour their lost child. When you lose a baby, you have a right to remember and honour that child in whatever way works for you. Grace confirmed that 'it's about having something tangible, somewhere to go, some way of remembering'.

We think of Lilly who sprayed a special perfume on baby Amilia Rose's blanket in the morgue and on her coffin.

And Maura who prays each night that she and her living children will be safe. In Maura's mind, her baby son Ronan is 'with [my] mother' who died many years ago.

Betty sets aside 'dedicated' time each week to sit and reflect on her son Joshua under the two big oak trees in the baby garden at Roselawn cemetery – a tranquil and peaceful space where she feels close to him.

John reminds us that lost babies are part of the family 'as much as any child who is walking around with you'. As the previous chapters have shown, parents have been on a huge emotional journey from the moment of conception … and we now come with open hearts to some of the tender moments recalled by the mums and dads.

'It is important that people acknowledge that your child was a person'

Recalling the first moment she saw Leonie Ellen's heartbeat on the scan, Tess said:

> From the first moment we saw her heartbeat she was our daughter, our child; still is and always will be … It is important that people acknowledge that your child was a person.

Bernadette too spoke of her baby being 'very present' to her when she saw the little heartbeat at the six-week scan. She thinks and talks about her five lost babies 'every single day' – losses that she thinks she may 'never be over'.

These sentiments are echoed in Beth's view that your baby 'is there in your heart forever … nobody has a right to tell you that you are wrong or you are over-exaggerating or whatever'.

Creating memories is paramount to many grieving parents. Every single moment of the journey with the baby is vividly documented and the tiniest detail matters to mums and dads.

As we will learn, the baby's memorabilia are forever cherished. These can include:

- a printout of a scan
- a photograph
- a footprint
- a handprint
- a lock of hair
- a little hat
- a teddy.

Drew, whose son Zach was stillborn at full term, recommended making memories in 'those first twenty-four hours'. He suggested bathing your baby, making sure your baby gets a name and taking as many photographs as possible.

In the pages ahead, parents share 'threads of enlightenment' for readers around the most precious and cherished memories of their babies. We learn that it can be highly emotional when the baby's memory box is initially presented; however, the box becomes a source of comfort, a treasure chest of memories as the years pass by.

'The most important piece of equipment you could get'

The memory box offered to bereaved parents by support organisations such as Sands and Féileacáin includes blankets, a teddy bear, a kit for little handprints, an envelope to store a lock of hair, and a disposable camera. John reckoned that the memory box is 'the most important piece of equipment you could get'. Framed pictures of his daughter Caoimhe's handprints and footprints taken after she was born adorn the wall at home. Interestingly, John suggested that parents might also consider keeping handprints of their living children, a practice which has become popular in more recent times.

For some parents it may be months or years before the memory box is opened – it is the parents' prerogative to do so when the time feels right. The consensus is, however, that it is 'invaluable' to have access to the memories, as they bring solace and comfort.

The following responses give us an insight into the importance and significance of the memory box for parents:

Lilly was delighted when the midwife presented her with a Sands memory box with a little white ribbon tied around it. She discovered that it already contained a photo of Amilia Rose, a teddy bear for Lilly to keep and one to put in the coffin.

Drew and Jo honour Zach's memory by opening the memory box to look at his footprints, handprints and photographs that they lovingly captured in the hours after his birth. Shauna too takes out her memory box around baby Branna's anniversary each year to look at photos, handprints and a precious lock of hair. She reads again the cards of support that people kindly sent. In the years that have passed since the loss, Shauna's husband has chosen not to look in the memory box. And that is fine too; the memory box is there for parents in whatever way they want to use it.

Mary loves that her memory box contains the little hat the nurses put on Emmet Pio the moment he was born. She imagines that she can still get the scent of him each time she opens the box. Maura cherishes Ronan's little knitted sleeping bag and the yellow blanket she kept in memory of him.

The importance of photographs and pictures

Many of us display photographs of deceased family members as a way of remembering and honouring those we love. Photos are also a significant and important way to immortalise the beautiful lives that could have been. A photograph can speak a thousand words: we may not need to say how we are feeling – we show the picture and that says it all.

Anna revealed her own profound psychological struggle with a framed photograph of her baby boy Gerry, born at thirty-two weeks. She was looking at his photo for three years before it 'dawned' on her that she was looking at 'the picture of a dead child'. She went on to say:

There was a day where the penny dropped – *that is a photograph of a dead baby*. I couldn't believe that I hadn't even registered it in my mind …

I was interested to know what the experience was like for Anna:

I just stepped back and thought, God isn't that odd having a photograph of somebody dead? I didn't want to think of it as being a photograph of a child that was dead – just a photograph of baby Gerry. It took me that long to even recognise that.

We know from studies that trauma can cause the body to be 'frozen' in time. In the presence of traumatic shock such as that experienced in stillbirth and miscarriage we 'preserve' ourselves from the overwhelming feelings by dissociating – in other words we 'disconnect' from our thoughts, feelings, memories and often surroundings too. Thinking about Anna and the sudden awareness of reality that came to her around the photograph of baby Gerry – we might say that Anna was, in that moment, coming out of dissociation and embodying feelings in the here and now.

We turn now to consider some of the huge decisions that parents had to make in the aftermath of their loss, a time when it might have been difficult to think clearly and to know what was best. For some, the need to honour their babies through baptism or wake was paramount.

The baptism, wake, funeral, cremation and grave

Mary and Lilly spoke of the importance of having their baby baptised in the hospital or at the wake that followed. Emily described Caoimhe's baptism as 'magical', surrounded by her loving family in the hospital. Parents had to decide whether or not to bring their child home to be waked. It is a deeply personal choice for each individual or family.

To have a wake or not

Maria made the choice not to bring Sam home as she was unsure how she might cope or how her children might react, as they were quite young at the time.

Mary's family supported her in waking Emmet Pio, which she deeply appreciated. The undertakers were waiting when she arrived from the hospital, and a little 'altar' of flowers and candles had been set up. The family accepted that at the time there was not a funeral mass for babies. However, the priest came and blessed the family before the burial at the cemetery.

Friends and family called to Tess's home to pay their respects, which 'turned into a wake'. It was important for them at the time that the parish priest was supportive and 'very much acknowledged' Leonie Ellen's existence. These are memories that are treasured forever. While it was 'tougher' to personally organise a funeral (rather than handing responsibility over to the hospital), it was, in the long run, the right decision for some.

Arranging a funeral

Drawing on valued advice he received when baby Zach died, Drew was clear that people should not live with regrets – instead have a funeral, give the baby a 'send-off', and organise a grave with your baby's name on it. However, arranging a funeral is a task that some people might not be able to contemplate. It is traumatic enough when an adult dies, but when the arrangements are put in place for a baby, it can feel unreal – 'how can this be happening?'

Maria decided to hold a private cremation with the help of the undertaker. Family members would have liked to attend, but Maria and Archie made the decision that it would be just the two of them.

While a service at the church for baby Amilia Rose was initially denied, Lilly and her partner David fought for her to be brought to the chapel for a service that included prayers and a little discussion. After David's friends sang 'Fields of Gold' and 'In the Arms of an Angel', David got up and spoke briefly – something Lilly was very proud of and a precious memory to hold on to.

At Caoimhe's funeral, those attending were instructed *not* to wear black. Emily wanted her baby celebrated and opted for butterfly blue and butterfly pink scarves for everybody to wear on the day. It was noted that the scarves were worn with 'such pride'.

A grave

In recognition of a baby's existence, a resting place is considered important. We are reminded by Maura and also by Leo that there is comfort in knowing where their respective children are buried so that they can go and visit the graves. Leo summed up his view:

It's much better to have somewhere you can go, a physical place … to pay your respects … a memorial to them … I thought it was very important at the time and still is.

How and when parents visit the grave of their baby is a personal decision. Some visit every Sunday and leave flowers, others save visits for special times such as Christmas, birthdays or anniversaries. It is heartening for parents when they go to the grave to discover that other family members have cleaned the headstone and laid flowers. A form of support that is noted and deeply appreciated.

Finding it 'too hard', Gretta rarely visits the grave where the names of her twins – Francis and Daniel – are etched on the headstone. Almost ten years have passed, yet the memories of the week in which she lost her second twin and lost her father are very clear in Gretta's mind, so much so, it's like 'it happened yesterday'. Interestingly, she expressed how she would love to make 'what's in [her] head into a film'. One interpretation of this is that Gretta's desire to project what is in her mind on to a screen is a need to release heavy emotions, perhaps as a way to observe feelings in a safe way from a distance, as it were. This book might also help to serve that purpose for readers.

Like Gretta, Drew does not go to Zach's grave to 'sit and grieve'. He prefers to keep busy and to 'spend a bit of time' with Zach through volunteering with the bereavement support organisation Sands. Some mums, like Cecilia, prefer to spend time 'talking' with their baby at the grave. At Christmas, as a way to 'include' Emmet Pio in the festival, Mary puts a tiny tree with a piece of fern on his grave.

However, visiting baby Gerry's grave on his anniversary is not easy for Anna and her husband Paul, or their children. Each journey in the seven-seater car is a reminder that there is an empty seat; that Gerry is not there. As Anna says:

You look at that seat and that seat is his. And that breaks my heart. If you are going on your holidays or going somewhere else, there is room … but there shouldn't be … because that seat should have been used.

Tess feels acknowledgement of her loss when the names of her three children are read out at the 'Blessing of the Graves' – an annual event in the Catholic church where families come to honour their loved ones and graves are sprinkled with holy water.

Kathy was happy that her four boys had their place of rest in their grandparents' plot – 'Angels Born Sleeping'. Serena too was happy to have her baby's 'little white box' blessed, wrapped in her mother's scarf and laid to rest in her grandmother's grave. Everyone brought flowers and walked with her to the graveyard – a treasured memory.

Babies' birthdays and anniversaries

Remembering babies' birthdays and anniversaries is also helpful and healing. Grace planted a cherry blossom tree in her mother's garden in memory of the first baby she lost. To honour Daniel, the twin who died, two little flowering shrubs were planted – both blossom at Easter time each year. Grace was angered though when two figurines of angels were stolen from the front step of her mother's house: 'The people who took them don't know the significance of them.'

Every 21 May on Alex's birthday, Cecilia and her family release balloons or tiny lanterns. They also planted a 'beautiful weeping willow' in their garden in her memory. When the family relocated, Alex's tree came with them – it was not going to be left behind!

Beth found the symbolism of planting a shrub in honour of her daughter to be affirming. She explained:

I bought a shrub and planted it in the garden … it took a while to be able to do it … she is there as part of our house and part of our home. When my children play in the garden, she's there.

After two 'hard years', Maria found contentment in knowing that Sam's ashes were at home with her, stored in a cuddle urn (the shape of a bear) and set in view on the fireplace. Wanting to find a meaningful way of remembering Sam, Archie took a tiny portion of the baby's ashes and had them mixed with ink for a tattoo. The timepiece clock tattooed on Archie's arm indicates the time of Sam's birth – it is 'a source of comfort and something that is there forever'.

When Sarrah phoned Sands she was greeted by a very understanding listener and was asked if she would like to bring a stone of her choice and place it in the Angel Garden for her daughter, Grace. Sarrah chose a grey washed-smooth stone and brought it with her. While painting the baby's name on it as well as three small flowers, and varnishing the stone with clear sparkly nail polish, she talked, and cried, and talked, in the presence of the listener who had taken her initial phone call. It was a welcome, healing encounter.

Both Ruth and her mother before her had the experience of losing a baby. Ruth's mother kept a little Christmas angel in memory of *her* lost baby whom she called John. In turn, she gave Ruth a little angel in honour of her lost child; something to keep for herself and feel that her 'baby is near'.

Marking the anniversary

Observing anniversaries is always a special way of commemorating those who have died. In some circumstances a decision has to be made about the most appropriate day to allocate as the anniversary.

Drew and Jo had to decide on which day to mark Zach's anniversary. In the end, 2 September (the day he died) was chosen. It is now a family day that they dedicate to him each year by taking the day off work.

Bernadette had a similar decision to make as her 'head was in a spin'. With five babies to remember and honour, she became 'fixated' on dates – the date of the miscarriage, the date the baby would have been born – to the point that it was 'getting like a compulsion'. In the end, it was relief all round when 24 April was selected as the date to remember all five babies. A little plaque in their memory and five little angels sit alongside family pictures in the sitting room.

Before bringing this chapter to a close, I would like to share part of Maura's story about her little son – a goosebump moment in the interview.

Talking to the 'wee boy'

Maura recalled that her son, aged two at the time, was down on his knees in the kitchen playing with his favourite little Fisher-Price toy. From the living room, the toddler could be heard chatting away, and this was not the first time Maura had witnessed this. She finally asked him, 'Who are you talking to?' He replied, 'The wee boy.' In that moment, Maura was stunned, but she firmly believes the 'wee boy' was the baby Ronan she had lost. She also draws comfort from the thought that Ronan is with her mother, who had died many years before. Due to her early death at forty-six, Maura's mother never got to meet her grandchildren. As such, Ronan is regarded as a 'gift', someone for her mum to care for and be a 'mother' to.

Reflection

This chapter contains deeply touching accounts of how lost babies are forever remembered and honoured. As the years go by, parents (and siblings) want to ensure that their baby – who, as Leo said, had a 'presence' in this world – is not forgotten. How this is achieved is the prerogative and personal choice of parents – it could be a shared experience, a memory or a 'sign' that brings peace of mind. In the end, it is whatever brings solace and comfort to the family that is important – whether the option is to open the memory box to recall and reflect, to visit the grave, plant a tree, have a tattoo inscribed, lay a painted stone in the angel garden, pray, take time for reflection, play a song, run a marathon to raise funds, organise a remembrance walk, or fast on Christmas Day.

We need to remember that bereaved parents can often be in the grip of powerful emotions. We do not always know what thoughts or feelings a mum or dad may be dealing with. So, let us not be judgemental; let us be respectful, compassionate and empathetic.

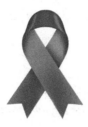

CHAPTER 10

'Men are not in the line of vision'

*The death of a baby impacts on people for the rest of their lives
... the smallest wee negative thing becomes huge
when you are in the pain of loss.*

Drew

*The sense of loss is momentous ... there is an ache for what you
have lost, an ache for what you have missed.*

Leo

Attempting to understand the complex emotional journey that often precipitates loss is critical to understanding how people grieve. Past research has indicated that men tend to rationalise grief and steer away from the emotional impact of loss. However, Bernadette McCreight's interviews with men attending pregnancy loss self-help groups contests this notion. McCreight found that males experience and deal with loss at an emotional level.

In this chapter we discover more about fathers' perspectives when the outlook for the baby is uncertain or when, sadly, miscarriage and stillbirth become a reality. Speaking openly and honestly from their hearts, fathers provided insights that enable us to learn more about the profound impact of the loss on men; how societal expectations almost demand that they remain, as Leo put it, the 'strong, durable person'; and that in essence, men can feel excluded, not included. The importance of dads being 'seen' and having a chance to express their grief is highlighted as a significant factor that can in turn determine the father's ability to offer emotional support to the mum.

Disregarding or excluding fathers can have far-reaching effects, as indicated in Willie's significant and important question: 'How can fathers be fully supportive if they are not recognised as bereaved and in grief?'

> I feel that excluding fathers is a way of further isolating the mother. That is, if a father is being treated like something outside the event, how could he be a support for his wife?

Perhaps in Willie's words there is good guidance not only for health professionals, but also for those in relationships and for society in general. It is clear that a sea-change is needed in attitudes towards men who are grieving. Willie continued:

> When a miscarriage occurs, men may revert back to the traditional male role that society appears to demand of them. This is often caricatured in such phrases as 'I heard your wife had a loss, here's a pint!' It is unacceptable, in some circles, for a man to claim any part of this tragedy as his own. Consequently, he can feel restricted and constrained in how he deals with the situation both introspectively and outwardly. This subsequently can adversely colour his reaction to the mother's sense of loss.

In essence, if the father is not 'seen' as part of the trauma of loss and cannot openly express his loss to others, the result may have far-reaching effects. Indeed, fathers may feel resentful that their feelings of loss are, as they perceive it, shut down by others. The 'silence' creates an internal emotional struggle which then impinges on the father's ability to comfort and respond to the mother who is grieving and in distress.

Therefore, Drew's statement that 'men are not in the line of vision' raises an urgent need for renewed attention to be given to fathers who may remain 'unseen' and unacknowledged in the circumstances surrounding the loss. As Leo put it, men may feel like 'an appendage; pushed to one side'. However, we learn that in the midst of the turmoil and trauma, dads do *not* want to remain 'unseen'. Rather, they want to be included, not excluded; acknowledged, not ignored.

'The loss is as equal for the male'

Core to the fathers' testimonies is a key message:

> the loss of a baby affects men just as deeply and as powerfully as it affects women.

Tony was clear that no matter at what stage the loss happens, it is 'enormous' for everybody concerned. The shock of Joshua's death was huge as Tony did not foresee that anything could go wrong. He felt 'no embarrassment or shame', however, in saying that when it comes to the trauma of the birth, 'Forget about the dad … first and foremost, the number one priority is always the mum'.

John too felt it was 'only right' that when his daughter was born, full attention was given to Emily and baby Caoimhe. He noted that if people did pay attention to him it was 'nearly an afterthought'. But he reiterated that men suffer as much as mothers do, particularly when the baby is born.

While the mum is in immediate need as regards medical attention, Leo reminds us that the 'father is there with her, worried about her, worried about the baby and worried about himself'. Leo considered that it might go back to societal expectations that the father is 'meant to be the strong, durable person' but added firmly that 'the loss is as equal for the male'.

Grace's own personal pain was so great that she 'couldn't see' the pain her partner was in, although she knew he was 'totally devastated'. The loss of their baby, she said, had such a 'massive impact on his life'. With no one else to talk to, Grace's partner found solace in speaking with *her* mum, someone he trusted – the grandmother of his baby. While Grace's dad saw all the suffering, like so many men he 'didn't know what to do or what to say'. He observed but did not share his feelings.

John pointed out that 'men by their nature don't open up as much as women' and that they need help to do so. In his view, now is the right time for men to move out of the traditional role; it is time now to change mindsets.

Drew noticed that there is a generation of men who will make small talk at wakes about cars and cutting the grass but do not necessarily talk openly about 'pregnancies, amniotic fluid and contractions'. He sees that society is changing, however, and he wants to ensure that men are informed, that they do not confuse loss as exclusively a woman's issue, or a failed pregnancy as meaning there is something wrong with the mother.

Let us stay with Drew's poignant account of his experience, which provides insight into the world of a father in an extremely traumatic situation. Three days before the birth, Drew and Jo became aware that Zach would be born without life:

You are standing looking on and Jo was bleeding uncontrollably and you start to read the signs from doctors – 'Can you bring blood on standby.' 'Can you get theatre ready, we need to control this bleeding.' At that stage I was standing holding Zach, who was dead, and … I thought was Jo going to die as well? So that process was long and extremely trau-matic … labour started on the Monday morning at nine and Zach wasn't born until forty-eight hours later on the Wednesday … inducement started to work and then didn't really work. Then it went to a different form of inducement and an epidural so it was a traumatic birth. Jo had severe lacerations that needed some stitches and surgery; she lost a lot of blood – she didn't need a transfusion but was on the verge of it.

Drew recalled that the midwife took Zach, put him in a cot and asked Drew to leave. He could not recall anyone asking him: 'How are you doing?'

Willie resonated with Drew's experience. 'It is very unusual … for anyone to ask the father: "How are you?"'

Indeed fathers may feel resentful that their feelings of loss, as they perceive it, are dismissed by others. Despite the lack of attention from others, fathers were very much 'seen' and firmly in the line of vision of wives and partners, as we are about to learn.

Men *are* in the line of vision

Some of the mums observed their men to be steadfast and courageous; others were aware that husbands and fathers felt helpless and unable to cope. We learn through the testimonies of mums how they welcomed and appreciated the sensitive and thoughtful support of partners and husbands. In the traumatic circumstances surrounding the loss of their baby, the impact of the loss on loved ones was 'visible' and never underestimated.

Many of the mums, including Ruth, Jane, Amy, Anna, Mary, Rose and Lilly, reflected on the emotional responses they witnessed, that remain etched in their hearts and minds. Recalling the scenes around the breaking of the traumatic news that their baby's health was compromised, and at the time of the births, they relayed how husbands and partners were distraught, crying hysterically, and how one dad 'went to pieces'.

Ruth's husband became 'very emotional' in the days following the loss of their baby at ten weeks. Serena felt that her husband 'took it worse' when the baby she was carrying was not visible at the fourteen-week scan. The loss retriggered the grief around his sister, a 9 lb baby, stillborn at full term.

Jane's husband 'always wanted children'. After the miscarriage he partly hid his own feelings in order to protect her:

> He was very supportive of me and he was upset for me. Was he upset for himself? If he was, he wouldn't have said it to me because he wouldn't want me to get upset.

Amy's husband was deeply upset when she miscarried four times. However, she recalled that he was 'just doing what men do in trying to hold it all together'. She notices however that when he hears of anyone having a miscarriage 'his heart sinks, and he feels really, really bad for them'. Clearly, news of a similar loss strikes at the heart of those who know the journey and know the pain it brings.

Anna recalled her husband Paul's face as 'ashen-grey' when the news of Gerry's death in her womb at thirty-two weeks was about to be confirmed:

It was just like somebody had torn him apart outside in … the realisation dropping on him …

And in quiet grief, Paul's colour did not return for some time:

Paul actually looked ghastly for months … he looked grey that whole winter and he would be quite silent.

Kathy, who sadly died before this book was completed, described her husband Ernest as 'heartbroken'. It hurt Kathy immensely watching her husband in tears holding baby Hyam, born at twenty-two weeks 'with his eyes open'. Ernest could see that the baby looked like him as they both shared the distinctive feature of a cleft on the chin. This was a touching, heartfelt moment that brought Kathy to tears in the interview and brought tears to me as well.

When they arrived at the hospital, Áine, who was in tremendous pain, recalled that her husband was 'sent away'. He did not know what to do or say and did not know how Áine was going to fare. The difficulty was that he did not have 'a support mechanism' as they had decided not to tell her husband's family about the loss. This was a decision that Áine, in hindsight, says 'may have been selfish' of her.

Wanting to make a difference, and remain in the line of vision!

In their desire to create memories, fathers made sure that they remained in the line of vision. Here are some of the touching accounts of making a difference and creating those precious memories.

Archie dressed, changed and photographed baby Sam. He made sure to get Sam's little hand print. Not only that, Archie held his baby son in his arms and was present in theatre while Maria had her placenta physically removed.

John 'stepped up' when Emily found that she was initially unable to take Caoimhe into her arms. He was 'delighted' and 'very proud' when he held his daughter.

Tony was very proud when his son was born: to him Joshua was not a dead baby. He proudly stated: 'He was our son.' Afterwards, Tony took on the supportive task of phoning family and friends, a role he considered as the traditional male role.

Phoning family and friends, however, was very difficult for Mary's husband Liam. He 'broke down' with each phone call.

While Tess was away getting stitches, her husband got to bathe and dress Leonie Ellen, the name he had already chosen for her.

Drew cut the cord and went on to wash and dress baby Zach. Knowing in his own mind that he was going to stay as strong as possible, Drew's focus was on Jo. He worried about how she would come through the loss of Zach and many questions were crossing his mind:

Imagine if Jo never recovers from this? What if she is the sort of person who goes into her shell and doesn't cope? What is the whole direction of life going to be now? We are very sociable people, we are very practical people, maybe we are going to lose all of this – is this the end of all of our happiness?

The reality was that Drew and Jo supported each other. On the days when Drew coped well, he supported Jo; other days Jo was stronger and supported Drew. It brought out the best in both of them – they were very determined that it was not going to be the end of all their happiness.

There are some things in life you cannot 'fix'

Drew described himself as a 'doer' and a 'fixer'. He acquired many books, read up about stillbirth and was 'going to fix the world' – find a solution in a month! As Drew learned, however, it all takes time, and when some things are fixed, new issues arise and some days are better than others. While calls for a dedicated midwife who is tasked with looking after bereaved parents is a valuable and important initiative that Drew is supporting within Sands, he also sees the need for home visits to support parents and to look out for mental health issues following a loss.

John and Willie also spoke of wanting to 'fix' things but discovered that there are some things in life you cannot fix. The desire to make things 'right' may be inherent, almost genetic, in men, John thought. When he and Emily learned that baby Caoimhe was seriously unwell and they made the important decision to go through the remaining seventeen weeks of pregnancy to full term, John slotted into a supporting role alongside Emily.

Willie had been willing to consider all options in their quest to have a baby, including IVF. He had been tense about the pregnancies but had resigned himself that if the treatment did not work, he and Catherine would 'deal with it'. As an adopted child, he understood the importance of having a child by any means possible:

> I am proof positive that the journey one undertakes to bring a child into a family becomes irrelevant when that child arrives. The first time that child cries for attention, you become the most important person in its life, and vice versa.

Men may 'run from it'

We have learned that men need support in their grief if they are to have the capacity to support their partners. While the feelings of bereaved fathers need to be validated and acknowledged, it has been noted that men may feel the need to 'supress' their emotions of grief and sadness in order to be strong for their partners. It could also be the case that they are lost as to what to do.

Feeling confused and vulnerable after losing her baby at eleven weeks, Gabrielle 'badly' needed the support of her husband. However, it was too painful, Gabrielle recalls:

> He [Gabrielle's husband] was so apart from me in the experience ... I had no one who had the strength to sit with me and process with me ... it was too painful for everyone. He ran from it.

The silence that followed the loss of Cecilia's baby Alex at sixteen weeks led in part to the breakup of the relationship. Efforts were made to keep the family together but the challenge was too great:

It still is tough, to be honest, now. My partner and I actually split up in the last year … he doesn't talk about it and I think … it has built up and built up and built up. He won't talk about it and he doesn't like me talking about it. He's had a lot of huge losses to contend with in his life … We did go to one counselling session but then he wouldn't go back … It was maybe about a month after we had lost her. I think maybe it was just too soon …

Here we see how the loss of baby Alex may have retriggered the grief of earlier losses in Cecilia's partner. We know that grief is a normal response to losing a loved one. However, if there are multiple losses over a period of time, the pain of loss can be overwhelming, especially if it remains internalised, not spoken about.

Tara noticed that her husband Michael went quiet and avoided talking about the two miscarriages she suffered. She interpreted the silence as perhaps his fear of upsetting her. Michael's philosophy is 'just let it be'.

Beth and her husband were on different wavelengths. While she felt she 'knew the baby' that she carried for eleven weeks, her husband did not understand where she was coming from. Later, when the baby was lost and flushed down the toilet, he struggled to recognise that it was a 'baby' that was flushed away – was it a baby or just tissue with blood in it? For the sake of peace Beth has decided to let it go and not talk about it, believing that to do so might not do either of them any good.

Eimear was surprised when her father, who would not normally display his emotions, commiserated with her when she lost her baby. Her husband did not view the loss in the same way, that is that it was an actual baby that was lost, at that early stage of pregnancy. In Eimear's view, the miscarriage did not have the same impact on him, or if it did, he did not show his feelings.

Reflection

A crucial point raised by Willie is that 'it is unacceptable, in some circles, for a man to claim any part of this *tragedy* as his own'. Fathers are in mourning yet societal expectations of denial seem to dominate when it comes to how others respond. And indeed, some fathers may welcome this as they may not wish to speak of the loss. While it may be argued that others are responding in the best way *they* know how or are comfortable with, there is a plea for a different approach.

The words of Matt Kahn, spiritual teacher and author, resonate with the plight of bereaved fathers when he says that people can only meet you as deeply as they have met themselves. Kahn's message suggests that the more we know ourselves – the more we are comfortable with and have addressed our own emotions – the more likely it is that we will feel at ease around people who are bereaved.

Another critical issue is this: if fathers have not had the chance to talk about the loss of their baby, not had the chance to express their grief and be supported, how can they in turn offer support to those around them who need it most – the mother of their baby, their wife or partner? Grief that remains inside can take a toll on mental, emotional and physical health. Feelings that are internalised cannot be seen but are, as it were, 'buried alive'.

Drew expresses movingly the situation in which men find themselves:

> I took time to say, *This is my grief time now*. The first Father's Day I said to Jo: 'I really need you to pick me up here.' The next time was actually the day before Zach's first anniversary. In my mind I was building towards that – I could feel the anniversary day coming … I was probably at my lowest, to a certain degree. I think men really need that space … I can remember just having this outpouring to my mum like I never had in my life before; just chatting to her and crying and it felt brilliant. It was so good. It was absolutely fantastic.

A final reflection

Fathers are asking for family, friends and society to allow them to talk:

- ask them about the baby;
- ask them about the loss;
- ask them how they are feeling;
- and be prepared to not only ask, but listen.

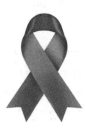

CHAPTER 11

'You lose a bit of yourself'

When you lose your child, you are fundamentally changed.

Sarrah

Losing a child is a lonely and personal grief because it was your relationship and no one else has the same relationship ... You can't share your grief with people because no one is grieving the same way. There is no sharing really ... sometimes even with your partner.

Leo

When the life of a baby comes to an untimely end at any stage from conception to birth, the depth and breadth of the emotional struggle that ensues is immeasurable. It is almost impossible to comprehend the rollercoaster of feelings that can be encountered in one hour, one day or one week when coping with the loss of the new life that expectant parents were waiting to welcome.

In this chapter, we are given privileged access to the raw, often 'unseen' emotions that losing a baby involves. Life is never quite the same again as many new and disturbing feelings erupt and have to be managed. As Tess said, 'When loss is suddenly at your door, you have to deal with it.'

Friends, as Tony and Betty found, can be a great support. After the funeral, however, when the rest of the world moves on, life stands still for bereaved parents. That is when despair and sadness kicks in. You, the reader, may 'see' yourself in the heartfelt experiences shared openly and honestly here.

Unless people have had the experience of losing a child, Leo said, they do not understand what it is like. The loss is personal and through it all, 'you lose a bit of yourself'. Grace agrees and asks people 'not to judge' as they may not fully understand if they have not suffered a miscarriage.

Maria expressed it in her way: 'After losing a child you will never be without pain.' However, she added that feeling pain is important as a marker that your baby is not forgotten and suggested that all anyone can do is 'learn to live around it'. In Sarrah's view, being bereaved of your child is the 'loneliest place in the world' because 'words are inadequate'. Beth still feels the emotional ache of the loss: '… something was taken away that belonged with us and we should have that human being'.

All of these accounts bring us into the personal turmoil suffered by the bereaved. The internal battle to comprehend the loss of the future and loss of potential – what could have been – is *one* of the most difficult aspects of this emotional journey. The painful part is that the answers to critical questions may never be known. You, the reader, may resonate with the important messages conveyed here as we explore the journey of loss.

The loss of what could have been: 'our future had now changed …'

We start with Drew's poignant recollection of a conversation with his wife Jo about the future without Zach:

> … it wasn't just Zach that died, it was our future – all his wee birthday parties, our Christmases, our holidays, grandkids, everything in our future had now changed. We

went through nine months adjusting our life to the fact that a baby was coming with the excitement building … and it was like a time bomb ready to go off … The stillbirth of a baby is the wrong way around … burying your child is not the way it is meant to happen.

Facing the future as a parent in mourning could not be more difficult. A situation can emerge that 'hits' like a bolt out of the blue and for some it can be almost unbearable. Few experiences bring home the pain of the loss as much as being in the presence of other people's children, encountering women who are pregnant or seeing babies that were born at the time that would have been your baby's birthday.

After her miscarriage, Eimear 'couldn't bear' to look at her husband nursing her sister-in-law's baby. She had to escape from the stress of the situation because of the emotions that flooded through her. She never explained to her husband how she felt.

Following the stillbirth of her son Joshua, Betty's emotional world was overtaken by thoughts of not wanting to touch babies, not wanting to hold babies or even to see anybody's baby. It was too painful. Her husband Tony suffered too. Anniversaries were difficult, while hearing crying babies or watching people push buggies set him off emotionally.

In the interview with Lilly I found myself gripped by her open and honest account, particularly when she shared her response to the news that a family member was pregnant. Lilly's feelings went into overdrive; in the end the pain was overwhelming:

It was awful. I hated her so much. All my family were congratulating her … I was jealous of her. It's okay to feel that way. I thought, *Why not her? Why did it have to be me? What have I done so bad in my life?* The night that she told me I went home and I got into Amilia Rose's cot, and lay and cried the whole night.

'There is that ache for what you have missed'

Mary was wistful for what could have been when she reached the landmark of four years since the loss of baby Emmet Pio:

> … seeing people that I knew were pregnant – you see their wee ones at nursery school, now getting ready for big school …

Witnessing the children of friends going through the different life stages stirred sadness in Leo. All the hopes and aspirations for his child who should have been going into secondary school had to be 'tempered':

> To never experience the joy of having that child, the fun … the hugs and kisses, throwing them on your shoulder … there is that ache for what you have missed.

Leo said the child remains 'present … an invisible person looking over your shoulder'. It's the expectation of the child and then 'coming home with nothing' that creates 'a higher magnitude of grief'. However, his other two children brought Leo comfort – a focus and a distraction. Part of the battle then was to look after the children, and reconnect with his work.

We turn now to another huge emotional hurdle that mums encounter in the days and weeks after the loss – the milk coming in.

'It was surreal'

When the milk comes in, so begins a period of yearning and longing, as Emily explained:

It was surreal … my body was still pregnant; my body had had a baby … and I was waking up on feeds, I genuinely was.

When Tess discovered her milk had come in she was upset, yet also found it 'comforting'. She felt like she was still 'a mammy' even though she did not have Leonie Ellen with her.

The milk coming in was difficult for Cecilia as it brought the loss back, raw. Having delivered baby Alex at twenty-three weeks, Cecilia was sad thinking that she should still be waiting on the birth, or at home breastfeeding a healthy baby. It took well over a year before Cecilia felt more 'like herself'.

In all of the poignant reflections above, we learn the truth of what can happen when emotional pain strikes at the core of a bereaved heart and mind. *Our* hearts and minds reach out in empathy and compassion. As the stories of loss continue, we learn more about the deep yearning, the residue of powerful emotions that continue to circulate in the internal world of the bereaved.

The what-ifs

As with many deaths and losses in life, the loss of a baby brings enduring what-ifs. Bereaved mums and dads can remain 'stuck' for many years as their minds wrestle with what could have been or what they could have done differently that might have saved their baby – a very painful and difficult place to be.

Maura 'analysed everything' as she relived the days and weeks prior to finding out that Ronan had died. The question loomed in her mind: '… was there something that I could have avoided that meant Ronan would be here with us today?'

What-ifs generate emotional disturbance and an ache inside. The ongoing internal battle can rob the bereaved of any opportunity for peace of mind. I was tearful as I listened to Lilly describe her first moments with her baby girl that are now embedded in her heart:

> I never got to know Amilia Rose. I will never know what she sounded like or how she cried; I have never seen her alive, I only knew Amilia Rose when she was dead. I would have loved to have heard her crying or just seen her moving or smiling. I didn't and I am not going to. It's hard.

Sarrah was left to wonder what Grace would have looked like. How she would have sounded. Her likes and dislikes. What she might have achieved at school. Would Grace have had 'mad curly hair' and inherited some of her dad's features?

Yearning and longing can sometimes be accompanied by additional powerful feelings, including guilt, jealousy and anger, well-documented responses to loss. Sometimes, it is generic anger at the world, anger at God, anger turned on

151

the self, anger with a partner or family or anger at the health professionals.

Inner hurt, anger and guilt ... 'What have we done to deserve this?'

Áine was incensed that she should suffer a miscarriage and recalled the pertinent question she launched out into the universe: 'What have we done to deserve this?' Having endured months of emotional turmoil following her husband's accident, the miscarriage was the last straw. However, Áine turned the anger inwards, attacking herself in the process:

> Why did my body do this whenever everybody else's body is perfectly capable of doing this? I was super fit ... at the gym four times a week ... two stone lighter ... I was so angry ... why could my body not grow a baby when everybody else is fit to do it ...?

The loss, still raw, left Áine wondering if the anger at *everything* would ever go away. Her strong feelings were exacerbated by the fact that her husband had children from a previous relationship that were unplanned and 'appeared as if by magic'. Áine wanted a baby so badly and wanted to prove that she could have a child. Amy too was 'bitter' with herself. She questioned why it had not happened for her and secretly harboured the thought: '... they are able to have a baby, why can't we have one?'

Tess felt pangs of guilt as she knew from before her marriage that her husband-to-be wanted children. She felt she was 'doing him an injustice' by not being able to provide the children he hoped for, although her husband acknowledged that it might be something to do with him. Tess had questions 'running around' in her head that 'friends and family could not see': 'Is it him? Is it me? Is it circumstance? What is it? Why has it not happened for us?'

Maria explained how she carried the emotional burden of guilt around baby Sam:

There's a lot of guilt, you know – my body has not kept Sam where he should be. I haven't kept him safe. I need to forgive myself.

Maria sought answers by attending a holistic therapist and having fertility massage, which focuses on improving circulation to the abdominal area. It can involve reflexology, acupressure, flower remedies, abdominal massage, pulsing, reiki, and the rebozo technique, which uses a shawl to massage the abdominal area in a gentle rocking motion.

From the perspective that the woman's womb and uterus are the centre of their energy, the therapist described Maria's womb as 'cold and sad'. I wondered what it was like to hear that feedback. Maria related to it on an emotional level; she visualised a 'dark, cold, empty cave'. In attempting to conceive again, everything the therapist recommended was tried, including hot castor oil compress packs on the lower abdominal area, massaging the womb area, positive affirmations, and so on. However, after losing the next pregnancy, Maria and Archie were emotionally and physically drained. They decided to stop trying for another baby. Maria thinks holistic therapy has a place in healing as it helped her tap into how her *body* was feeling.

Around the time of the loss of Ellen at thirty-eight weeks, Rose found patience hard to come by. She feels much angrier now than at any previous time in her life. It was helpful that the consultant suggested that Rose need not forget about Ellen but perhaps 'park' her loss before embarking on another pregnancy; his 'kind and lovely manner' enabled her to accept his guidance.

Emily's anger arose as she absorbed the difficult news received at the hospital. The consultant was clear that should Caoimhe live, she would have to be moved immediately to another hospital. If this were to happen, John could go with Caoimhe but not Emily. Such was the extent of the all-consuming anger she felt on the journey home, Emily contemplated getting out of the car and walking. She just wanted 'out of there'.

At the funeral of the mother of a colleague, Beth watched people crying at the graveside and felt a mixture of jealousy tinged with anger. She did not have the same opportunity to honour her baby and wondered to herself:

Why can others grieve a loved one and I can't grieve my baby? ... I couldn't grieve openly ... I couldn't wear black and have a wake and a funeral.

As Beth continued with her story, I could feel anger rising within me as I listened to the comments that had been directed at her:

'Don't be so sad';
'Pull up your socks and go back to your life';
'At least you have a baby; there are some people who will never have a baby'.

Consequently, Beth felt unable to open up and be honest about how she was feeling; it also left her questioning if it was 'ridiculous' that she named her baby, bought a shrub and planted it in the garden in Grace's honour. I find myself wondering how you, the reader, feel about Beth's experience.

Suicidal thoughts and depression

Sarrah noted how fundamentally people are changed by the loss of a child and how hard the emotional fall-out can be. At her lowest point following the loss of Grace at twelve weeks, she contemplated suicide:

> When you lose your child you are fundamentally changed; on some level you are mad: 'If I die ... Grace won't be on her own, I'll be with her'.

While she actively made preparations – with tablets, milk, photos of her children and a suicide note – she fortuitously realised before it was too late that she would only be 'handing down' her pain, especially to her daughter, who would be the one to come through the door and find her. That realisation was a turning point. Instead, Sarrah became involved with helping other people in a similar situation, something she sees as giving her life a purpose.

Tess would not consider suicide as she holds the view that her losses are 'God's will'. In her mind, if she took her own life, she would not get to heaven and in the afterlife would not get to meet with Leonie Ellen, Leo and Dylan. The possibility of a 'reunion' has kept Tess going.

Bridget's many miscarriages and an ectopic pregnancy took a toll on her mental health. She became severely depressed such was the level of grief she was going through. She explained:

I didn't want to get out of bed. I didn't want to sleep. I didn't want to eat. You just go from one extreme to the next and drink was a very close comfort for me. If I hadn't had the support … I have no doubt that I would have gone down the drink road … because nobody understood.

The emotional and physical reactions to the trauma of stillbirth and miscarriage can infuse the bereaved mind with panic, fearfulness and anxiety. This emotional fall-out can impact on almost every aspect of life as the trauma of loss can take a huge toll. While the well-being of many bereaved parents may not be affected in the way described below, it is useful to learn about the experiences shared in the interviews:

Reluctant to leave the children

Amy has found it very difficult to trust anyone with her children, other than her husband, mother and childminder. She is reluctant to leave the children or be away from them, especially at night. If she does surrender to going out, she just worries 'so there is no point'. While at work, Amy is reassured by the knowledge that her children are well cared for by her childminder, to whom she paid credit:

It's a testament to her that I don't think about them during the day because I know she is minding them … putting sun cream on them …

Stuck in a particular state of mind

Ruth is afraid of going out in the car with her children, a phenomenon that has developed since she lost her baby. She lives in fear of an accident that would be her fault, in which she might lose one or all of the children. Ruth recognises that having such fear is 'not right'; a state of mind where she sees herself as stuck, not having 'moved on'.

'The most horrendous experience ever'

Following the loss of Emmet Pio, which Mary described as 'the most horrendous experience ever', she 'kept getting this notion' that *she* might die and leave her living children without a mother. Emmet Pio's death brought her face to face with her own mortality.

'Somebody was going to come in and take him away'

In Lilly's psyche the loss of her daughter was deep-rooted. Trust was hard to come by. The arrival of a new baby boy did not prevent intense fears and worries:

> I was convinced, now that we had a healthy baby at home … that something was going to happen or somebody was going to come in and take him away.

This extreme anxiety was also what Maria experienced in the weeks and months after Sam died. She too feared that something was going to happen to her other children:

- She felt as if she was not in control of her emotions.

- She did not want to go out.

- She did not want to meet anybody.

- She actively avoided people.

- She became hyper-vigilant and would not let her son out of her sight.

So intense was her worry that she had 'actual visions of him being knocked down'. The anxiety remains with her and has transferred to other situations, including driving her car and her eldest son leaving home.

Reflection

The deeply touching, open and honest accounts in this chapter bring home explicitly the rollercoaster that life becomes in the aftermath of the loss of a baby. Feelings and emotions are highly charged and there is much for mums and dads to cope with as they make their way through the unpredictable emotional terrain that seeps into every aspect of life beyond loss. It is almost as if this chapter needs to be read again and again to allow us to fully grasp the extent of what has been termed 'the loneliest place in the world' and to understand that when you come to that place in life 'you lose a bit of yourself'.

Before completing this chapter and this reflection I want to bring you back to an experience that Anna shared openly. Anna's baby Gerry was stillborn at thirty-two weeks and later she became pregnant again. Here Anna describes the feelings and emotions around the arrival of baby Patrick, born with Down's syndrome and a heart defect:

> Going back to that day we left the hospital, we were taking what we got and thanking God for it but we knew it would be a different journey than with the other kids at home. A heart defect and Down's syndrome wasn't what we were expecting in our new baby but he was alive and we were delighted. There was a knot of anxiousness about the heart condition and about the level of abilities that he would or would not have. It wasn't the same feelings of unblemished joy that I had leaving the hospital with the other three. There was a sadness that life would be hard for him, and, if I'm honest, hard for me trying to manage his abilities (how silly that seems now with hindsight). But it was 'king' compared to the feelings of utter devastation of leaving with no baby.
>
> We had been to the opposite end of not taking home a baby and were delighted now to take home a breathing baby, appreciating a child that was alive even with all the unknowns and worries that lay ahead – we were ready to take on whatever came.
>
> Patrick will soon be ten years old. Goodness, when we left the hospital with a child that had Down's syndrome and a heart defect we were terrified that maybe he wouldn't live long. Patrick's as healthy as a trout now and had a heart operation when he was three.

From Anna's experience we learn that, in losing a bit of yourself through pain and suffering, you can also gain perspective and resilience that sets you up for whatever lies ahead.

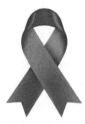

CHAPTER 12

Finding a 'Saviour'

*Grief taught me to get to know the new me because I could
never be the same again …*

Emily

Over the years as a volunteer with Cruse Bereavement
Care, I have sat with many bereaved people struggling to come to terms with the loss of a loved one.
The 'work' of bereavement counselling is to help people begin
to understand *who they are* beyond the loss that has changed
their lives forever. It is the beginning of an uncertain journey,
and if we are on that journey, we are unsure where the creation
of a 'new me' will lead us to, how we will get through it or how
long it will take. Emily explained:

> Grief taught me to get to know the new me because I could
> never be the same again … I had to sit with feelings that
> I didn't know existed … didn't know what they meant;
> reactions that I didn't know were possible … it's a permanent
> journey and permanent learning

We know that the journey through grief and mourning is personal, and is different for each individual. It is the *relationship*
with the deceased that determines the nature of the challenge
ahead. Psychological research into loss has shown that the
closer and more meaningful the relationship, the tougher the
journey beyond the loss.

It is known that being listened to and 'heard' can help
the bereaved process loss and grief. When people grasp
the opportunity to avail of bereavement counselling, they
sometimes speak of it as a 'life-saver'. What this really means

is that the person is their own saviour. Investing time in counselling opens up the opportunity to gain greater insight and understanding of self; generating a level of acceptance, and hope for the future.

We discover here that bereaved mums and dads were determined in their efforts to find a way through the quagmire, the avalanche of emotions and pain-provoking situations that they faced in the weeks, months and years after the loss of their baby. As we are about to learn, the 'saviour' appeared through different avenues. We begin with Lilly's powerful and poignant story of finding salvation in the most unexpected place.

'She listened to me. It was all I needed'

In the depth of grief for her daughter Amilia Rose, Lilly began to drink – not to get drunk, but 'to stop feeling so shitty' and to numb the pain of loss:

> That awful feeling inside. That sickening feeling. You feel numb. You don't know what you feel. You can't feel your heart beating. I was so lost in my grief … I did not want to be alive anymore. I wanted to be dead.

Lilly did not think she would find her 'saviour' at the graveside of her baby girl. For three months she regularly sat at the grave for hours:

> I just stayed at the grave all the time, I didn't want to leave her, I felt really bad for leaving her … You get crazy … I said

to David [her partner] what happens if she starts crying? It could be raining and I could just have been sitting at the grave and no coat on me and me soaking wet. I was never aware of what was going on around me ... sitting maybe in wet clothes for hours. I didn't even know it was raining; couldn't have told you what it was doing ...

Buried alongside Amilia Rose was a young woman who had died of cancer at the age of twenty-four. Her mother attended the grave regularly and, in the end, she was the person who gave Lilly hope and saved her life:

She sat with me so many times in that graveyard in the rain and she never said, 'Come on, let's go, come on, Lilly.' She sat and she talked to me and she listened to me. It was all I needed. We are great friends now. Only for her I don't think I would be here, I would be probably dead now, I know that. When she is feeling down on the anniversary of her daughter I give her hope and I keep her going.

Lilly gained perspective and empathy. She recognised that she had lost her baby but also learned about the pain of losing an adult child – a pain, she said, she would never want to imagine. Later she added that Amilia Rose's death had taught her not to be selfish, and to listen. She wanted to be a better human being and to *really* listen to others.

The message coming through is critical for all to hear: bereaved parents *need* space and an opportunity to talk, someone who will listen with no judgement and no pressure.

Don't let it be the 'elephant in the room'

Determined not to allow the loss of baby Gerry to be the 'elephant in the room', Anna created her own saviour. She took the courageous step of calling into her local shops on the way home from the hospital and informing everybody about the loss of baby Gerry. The risk of people not knowing about her loss would have resulted in the 'inevitable' question: 'What did you have?' Anna opened up to those who did not know what to say. In her view, the loss had happened; it needed to be talked about and she needed to protect herself from the pain of innocent inquiry.

Tess and her husband talk about Leonie Ellen all the time. However, feeling comfortable in talking is the 'biggest thing':

> You have got your friends and family and you nearly know who you can talk to and who you can't because you know by their reaction ...

While John and Emily welcomed the opportunity to speak publicly about their loss and agreed to be interviewed on national television, others like Leo and Gretta were reluctant to talk about their bereavement. Gretta was clear that 'it is not the sort of thing you would talk to friends about'. The interview for the book was 'the longest conversation' she had had. Leo thought that getting 'involved' in someone else's loss might 're-ignite a deep sense of your own loss which you have dampened down with time ... it's not like you take some tablets or get an operation, and it disappears'.

Returning to work: how and when

The decision to return to work after the loss of a child can be a difficult one. Going back can have mixed blessings: for some, work became an additional challenge; for others it was a 'saving grace', a chance to 'feel normal'.

Finding a way to cope with the onslaught of emotions that arise can be a huge challenge. What becomes clear is that, while people in the workplace may not want to mention it, there are bereaved parents who would prefer that the loss is recognised and validated, as a lack of acknowledgement creates an anger inside. In essence, if others are worried about bringing up the loss of a baby, the message from parents is clear: bring it up, and let the parents decide how they wish to respond.

When Maria returned to her teaching role after losing baby Sam, it felt like she was 'laid bare and exposed'; as a result, she was very angry. People seemed to ignore her loss but could openly talk about other losses – and it hurt, even though she knew they were scared of 'saying the wrong thing':

> Going in to school I felt the anxiety – you are just laid bare – everything is so raw and open and I think with any other type of death people will ask ... but a baby death they don't want to talk about; they don't want to bring it up and they don't want to say anything because they are afraid of saying the wrong thing. And then it's the elephant in the room – nobody will speak about it.

The loss of Sam created 'unseen' sensitivity. Most frustrating of all was observing others in the school having the 'freedom' to speak about their loss – other types of bereavement – and openly share stories and pictures. The parent who apologised to Maria for being late for a parent–teacher meeting due to the demands of her baby's feeds was not intended to hurt. But it did hurt, deeply.

Gretta felt differently. When she contacted her head of school with a view to returning to her post, she was surprised with the level of support offered to her. While she recognised that colleagues were lovely, kind people, she also knew that she 'couldn't cope' if they mentioned the baby. Her response would be 'unpredictable' and 'breaking down in tears' was not something Gretta wanted to happen. She managed the situation by emailing ahead, asking that the staff would be informed in advance of her wishes. Interestingly, it was on her return to work that Gretta found herself thinking more about her loss even though she tried hard to block it all out.

Sarrah's experience was different again. Within a few days of her loss, she decided to go back to work. However, she felt like a 'wind-up doll'. That is, she 'wound herself up' to be able to go to work, covered up her quietness in front of colleagues with the excuse of a headache, and then came home and had a 'meltdown'. We can only imagine how strenuous it is to manage such an emotional rollercoaster.

Tess, on the other hand, welcomed the opportunity to 'go back to work and be normal'. Not using her brain left her 'thinking too much'. So, returning to work was part of her saving grace at the time.

Áine, however, offered a warning to those bereaved of a baby not to return to work too soon. She put herself under pressure to return at a particular time of the year, and as she looks back she recalls that 'it was a blur'. Physically she was sore and mentally she was in a 'state of disbelief' after everything she had been through. Áine's message was clear – wait until you are ready.

'Live in the present'

Emily's 'miracle baby', Caoimhe, taught her to live in the here and now. In response to those who ask her: if she could go back, change things and wipe it all out, would she do that, Emily's answer is clear: 'Absolutely no way, no way'.

> Caoimhe taught me to very much live in the present. Because that is all I had. She taught me to not go further because to go further was too painful; to even think to go further was going to rob me of the time that I had with her.

One of Drew's 'saviours' is his faith, which he describes as 're-ally important' to him as he and Jo are steeped in church life. In the aftermath of their loss, their faith became even more important. Drew was brought up in the belief that when ba-bies die, they go to heaven. Drew believes that Zach is in heav-en, at peace and at rest. On the day of the baby's funeral, he and Jo had an 'overwhelming' sense of peace, something never felt before. A decision they made was to find a way to laugh again someday, something they regarded as 'a really good am-bition to have'. In seeking help and support from the church congregation, Drew and Jo said there were people who came 'out of the woodwork', saying, 'you probably never knew this, but it happened to me'. They had lost babies thirty and forty years ago.

At the time of her loss, Serena felt buoyed by her belief and philosophy that 'souls are recycled' and 'it just wasn't the right time' for her baby. However, she was acutely aware that the loss of a baby can impact across the generations. Many years previously her mother-in-law had suffered loss through stillbirth. She rarely spoke about it but it took a huge toll on her mental health. At the birth of Serena's three daughters, her mother-in-law became depressed for months. Here we learn again about the impact of grieving in silence with little emotional outlet. Serena felt sorry for her mother-in-law and recognises now that had she, Serena, gone full term and ended up giving birth to a fully formed baby that had died in her womb, she 'wouldn't have been able to deal with it'.

The 'secret club' that you don't want to join, but …

Tony described Sands (stillbirth and neonatal death support charity) as the 'secret club' that you don't want to sign up for, yet both he and Betty are adamant that they could not have made it through without the organisation's help. Betty, now a trained befriender, said the key is that you meet people who 'know exactly' what you are going through, and added that 'speaking out' helped to cement her and Tony's relationship:

Emotionally and psychologically our relationship grew stronger, we bonded together a lot closer.

Betty recognised that she and Tony dealt with their grief differently. As the months went on, they tentatively investigated the possibility of help through Sands. It was arranged that they would first meet with a 'befriender' who was able to reassure them that Sands was a place where they could choose how to talk – or not! As it turned out, they found the courage to 'open up more'. Betty explained:

> We surprisingly ended up talking and very much told our whole story. I think I realised that it really helped me to talk – it made him [Joshua] feel like he was real ... there is this perception that if he was never here, he didn't really exist.

Tess too endorsed Sands: '... you feel like you are not going insane. You are not crazy, you are not mad. And that it's okay to talk about it'.

The saviour for Maria was Cruse Bereavement Care. At her first session she 'just went in and cried, just cried, couldn't really speak'. Six sessions spread over a number of weeks brought about a healthy change. In the lead-up to Christmas that year Maria was 'able to go in and talk and laugh with the counsellor', who recognised how far she had come.

Bridget sought help through counselling but found that it did not help. She and her partner got through it all themselves. However, she feels lucky to have been signposted by the fertility network to support groups that work hand-in-hand: IVF and miscarriage support groups.

Tess wanted to alert readers to a charity called Count the Kicks that educates women and raises awareness about the kicks of the baby. With her first pregnancy, Tess recalled there was very little talk about baby movements. She now finds it consoling that progress has been made and that there are more indicators of what can go wrong.

The 'saviour' found in fundraising

Part of Drew's coping strategy was to focus on fundraising for Sands, which he described as his 'release'. The funds raised supported the development of a bereavement suite at the local hospital. The aim was to create a 'less clinical and more comfortable environment in which to create memories for people who are grieving'. Drew continues to raise funds, which helps to raise awareness:

Stillbirth happens and we need to look out for vital signs.

Maria too wanted to raise funds for Sands. Her husband Archie ran a marathon; and she and her sister-in-law did a 5K and also raised funds with a non-uniform day in her school – all in honour of the four children she lost.

In 2016, Bernadette set up a miscarriage support group in Galway. At meetings of the Miscarriage Association of Ireland where she volunteers, she still finds herself upset when talking about her experiences, even though many years have passed. Reflecting on her losses, Bernadette said: 'They are part of my history … and made me who I am today.' She organises an annual remembrance walk to raise funds, and explained that an elderly man joined them on the last walk. He told Bernadette that his deceased wife had lost a baby many years ago and he wanted to honour her memory and honour their baby by joining the walk. A deeply touching account and a reminder that indeed the loss of a baby is carried forever.

Supporting 'the slow release of grief'

Becoming fully fledged members of a Féileacáin bereavement group enabled both John and Emily not only to be helped personally, but in turn to help others. At various events organised by Féileacáin, John has witnessed 'rooms full of people … there for the same reason'. John and Emily have hosted events in their city and continue to meet an enormous number of people seeking support. Rose too benefited through the help she received at a Féileacáin bereavement group, which she described as 'amazing'.

John explained how Féileacáin was contacted by thousands of people – many bereaved long ago – after an episode of *Coronation Street* was aired. Kym Marsh played the part of a woman who had lost a baby at twenty-four weeks. Ironically, the actress herself had lost a baby at an advanced stage of pregnancy many years before, a personal loss she spoke about courageously at the time of the *Coronation Street* episode. Féileacáin and TV3 (as it was then) wanted to make a response to those whose memories of loss and grief were retriggered. John and Emily agreed to take part in a television interview to tell their story. The response from the public was 'huge': people wanting to tell their own stories and praising the couple for how they dealt with their loss. John believes that it's about Caoimhe:

As time has gone on, Caoimhe has taught us so much; as a family we have been so lucky, it has brought us together … she has taken us to some amazing people and amazing places …

Reflection

At the start of the chapter Emily said that grief had taught her to get to know 'the new me' as life would never be the same again. We know that the journey beyond loss is not easy and indeed is never the same again. We know that those who sought out help through Sands, Féileacáin, Cruse Bereavement Care and other organisations had an outcome that was greater than might ever have been expected.

For some, the stress of loss on the body and on the emotions continues to impact in daily life. Others discovered a 'saviour' in the most unexpected places. We can only admire the strength, courage, openness and honesty of all the contributors who have helped us learn about the true meaning of stillbirth and miscarriage in their lives.

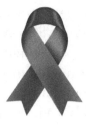

Final Reflection

Dear Reader

As I begin to reflect on this precious book, *Stillbirth and Miscarriage, a Life-changing Loss: 'Say my baby's name'*, my thoughts turn to the journey that the bereaved parents and I have been on over the past number of years. It is one of the greatest privileges of my life to share this journey with the parents who have contributed so kindly and generously to make this book possible. I am very proud of what we have achieved together and I think that my mam would be equally proud that we, with the kind help and guidance of Dr Marie Murray, the editor, have brought this book to fruition.

The book would not have been created without the willingness of you, the parents, to give the 'gifts' of your time, your voices, your history, and your legacy of loss. Our deepest thanks are due to the five dads and twenty-seven mums who provided memorable and deeply touching insights, and much food for thought. We can only admire your strength, openness and honesty in this quest to know and understand the true meaning of the life-changing losses that are stillbirth and miscarriage.

My thoughts now turn back to my mam and to Patrick, her third child, that she referred to as her dead-born son. Her grief was carried in silence and yet it was etched on her face and in her demeanour. Patrick was born in an era where such losses were rarely spoken about. Perhaps people were afraid to ask in case the wounds of the loss were reopened or they felt that they could not cope in such a sensitive situation. I am thankful now and cherish those moments when Mam spoke about Patrick; she told me in her own words and with her own voice what happened in those last weeks of her pregnancy and how Patrick was taken away in a shoe-box to be buried. It is also somewhat gratifying too that when the priest reassured her that Patrick would indeed have been baptised through 'baptism of the will', Mam finally found a degree of peace and comfort – small mercies in a difficult life journey beyond a loss that was grieved in relative silence.

Mam would appreciate and understand the need to give voice to the loss that profoundly changes people's lives, as many parents know only too well. The legacy of the loss is carried forever and it is important to say that this book honours and is mindful of *all* those who have lost their beloved baby.

Now that the book is complete and ready to go out into the world, I feel a level of personal contentment. The responsibility of managing the sacred testimonies through the journey from interviews to the finished book has been 'living' in me since the study began. I carried the work in my heart and in my head every step of the way. It is gratifying that the babies who are no longer with us are remembered, acknowledged, validated and respected.

We know that we are following in the footsteps of previous research papers and books that have enlightened and 'educated' us all. Let us hope that this book keeps the light around stillbirth and miscarriage burning brightly so that we will pay attention more consciously and mindfully to those who suffer the loss of a baby through stillbirth and miscarriage.

May all of you who are reading this book in the hope of easing your own pain find solace, comfort and healing through each of the chapters.

With love, regard and respect,

Anne

Dialogue with the Healthcare System

Important developments in relation to stillbirth and miscarriage in recent years include firstly the provision of bereavement suites in hospital settings. In conjunction with the suites, childbirth and pregnancy loss specialist midwives have been assigned in some trusts in Northern Ireland. Similarly, in the Republic of Ireland, pregnancy loss midwives have been appointed in many of the maternity units. Following the publication of the *National Standards for Bereavement Care*, hospitals set up groups to oversee the implementation of the standards. In relation to those in same-sex relationships who have suffered the loss of a baby, important changes have been introduced to the literature.

Carole McKeeman, the Western Trust bereavement coordinator, kindly highlighted a critically important addition to the information issued by the Miscarriage Association. The footnote states:

> This leaflet is for *all* partners of women who have miscarried. This includes lesbian, bisexual and transgender partners. We recognise that some readers may no longer be with their partner, but we hope this leaflet is still helpful.

Thank you, my dear friend Carole, for sharing this important addition.

Melissa Crockett, one of the first specialist midwives in the Western Trust, developed the idea of a football team for dads, brothers, nephews and any other men affected by baby loss. Consequently, in collaboration with Sands, the NI Maiden City football team was founded. The idea is to provide a resource for men, grieving the loss of a baby, to come together in a supportive environment where they can play football and choose to talk or not talk!

A similar endeavour is underway through Féileacáin, headed up by Ken Walsh, Tony Owens and Anthony Casey in Ireland. Monthly training sessions were planned, as well as a special fundraising football match in May 2020. Bereaved fathers were to sport a football jersey with their child's name on it. In an interview in 2020 with Louise McSharry of 2FM in Dublin, Ken noted the alarming statistic that Féileacáin provided almost 900 memory boxes to hospitals in 2019. The need for help and support is ongoing.

Without question, a Birth Acknowledgement Certificate or Certificate of Life are welcome and important developments to honour babies who have died, lost through stillbirth or miscarriage. Healthcare professionals will now be aware of the five types of certificates available, depending on the circumstances.

We are more aware than ever of the heartfelt experiences and enduring sense of loss that is the legacy of stillbirth and miscarriage. Now, bereaved parents wish to address health professionals, other bereaved parents, society in general and religious organisations to raise awareness:

AWARENESS FOR HEALTH PROFESSIONALS

- **Bereavement training** should be 'mandatory' for all

- **Be careful in the use of language around mothers**
  Terms such as 'tissue', 'evacuation', 'abortion' or 'spontaneous

abortion' are considered 'harsh' words for what is a very personal type of procedure.

- **'The stillborn down in room 10'**
  Please know that this is devastating for a mother to hear. Her child is 'no longer a person, just a stillborn' but to her the child was her life and was going to be a big part of her future.

- **'What do you want us to do with the remains? Do you want us to dispose of them?'**
  Bereaved parents do not welcome questions posed in this way.

- **'Please don't be clinical'** … when telling mothers and fathers the news that all is not well with their baby. Remember it is not 'clinical' for them.

- **Less medical, more caring….**
  'If my experience had been a bit more caring it would have allowed me to be a bit more caring with myself.'

UNWELCOME MESSAGES 'STICK'

'You are lucky, you have four lovely children and you are young … if this is the worst thing that happens to you, you will be okay.'
  Please know for many parents '*it is* the worst thing that has ever happened'.

'Go home and try again when you are ready.'
  'That is not what you want to hear at that time.'

'One of those things'
  'It was pretty much brushed under the carpet by the doctors

– one of those things that happens and very common in first pregnancy.'

'Whatever was there has gone.'

'… [the nurse] scanned me and said, "oh sure there is nothing there; whatever was there has gone". … no skills … I can still see her face today'.

'You should have gone to the toilet before you came down here'.

'The nurse was very abrupt. I was on the toilet before I buzzed … that always stuck in my head … she was rude.'

'Your baby is dead.'

'A doctor came in … quite abrupt … he started to scan me … he said, "Your baby is dead … there is no fluid." He took the scanner away, left my baby on the screen and walked out of the room.'

'He was completely dismissive of everything'

'The doctor came round, I hadn't seen him before … he was completely dismissive of everything … he came with the wrong file … and asked me about having a fit … that wasn't me.'

Keep mothers separate

'I was put in a ward full of women … in for bedrest; their babies were healthy. I was stuck in this ward and I knew ours was dying … hearing all these conversations … what they were having and the names that they'd picked; I'm sitting there … what was I going to talk about?'

GOOD MESSAGES ALSO 'STICK'

'He understood'

'[the doctor] put his hand on my hand and he was almost emotional … he understood, you know … he genuinely was concerned …'

'She was holding my hand'

'One of the midwives who was there when they had to take the placenta away was very encouraging … the whole time she was holding my hand … and saying to me you can do it – you are nearly there and she was very good. Her name was … the same as Mummy's.'

'Life is a miracle …'

'A young doctor came round and he says, "I do at least one or two of these procedures every day … so … life is a miracle, life is precious." He explained it so nice and he was so lovely.'

'[The midwife] treated everything with dignity …'

'The sister who ended up delivering Amilia Rose treated everything with dignity, she was respectful and she was professional and so empathic.'

'Don't worry, pet, it will be okay'

'I just remember a nurse holding my hand a lot of the time. I just cried and cried. And she told me, "Don't worry, pet it will be okay."'

'Our nursing experience was excellent'

'I had heard horror stories from other people; real disaster stories about treatment, the wrong words and the wrong things but … our nursing experience was excellent … concern and compassion … if I meet the person I say, "You are the midwife who was there for us."'

TIME TO 'INFORM' THE HEALTHCARE SYSTEM

- **Don't run away and hide** or get another medical professional – please say, 'I'm really sorry about the baby.'

- **'You just need your little bubble'**
  It is 'cruel' to be put in a ward alongside a mother with a new-born baby crying. A bereavement suite that is soundproofed would be ideal – 'you just need your little bubble … no matter what other room you go into you are going to resent it'.

- **The 12 o'clock appointment**
  Parents want to be more than a number on a list.

- **No false hope**
  The medical profession should not give false hope by saying, *I know somebody else who had bleeding right throughout the pregnancy.*

  'Deal with me and tell me what exactly is happening with *my* body.'

- **If a procedure such as a stitch is needed to save the baby—** make sure it is not overlooked or put on hold (if more than one hospital is involved in the care of the mother).

- **Incorrectly recorded** medical notes are deeply upsetting, especially if, for example, postpartum psychosis instead of postpartum depression is recorded in the file.

- **The Sands sticker**, a 'warning' of a previous stillbirth, is on the front of the patient's file. It includes the baby's name and date of birth. Paying attention to it would ensure that bereaved parents are not asked over and over – 'Is this your first baby?'

- Be 'caring and understanding' of what a parent is going through.

- 'More empathy needed for parents and families'.

- **'Don't forget the human being'** who is struggling, overwhelmed with feelings and hormones; it's an 'unpredictable' place to be.

- **Talk through what is going to happen** during the labour. Parents need 'warning' of what to expect, especially 'the silence in the room' following a stillbirth.

- **'Miscarriage is a taboo subject'** – even in the hospital. Nurses are busy and don't have time to talk. But parents may need 'direction', particularly after two miscarriages ... seeking help through a specialised clinic, for example.

- **'Early pregnancy loss'** is a better expression than miscarriage. 'Where is the baby in miscarriage?'

- **A mothers needs reassurance** that miscarriage does not mean the end of her chances of becoming a mum. Please respond kindly to significant questions: 'Will I ever become a mother?' 'Was it something I did that caused this to happen?' 'Is this going to happen again?'

- **Parents need choice**

  Explain the choices and let mums and dads decide the following:

  – how and in what way they wish to go from the delivery suite to the ward with their stillborn baby;

  – how they wish to leave the hospital – a critical issue as bereaved parents are deeply sensitive in the situation:

  'Don't ask us to leave the hospital through the pregnancy admissions area. Unless we choose to.'

  While probably well intentioned, offering parents the choice to leave by a different exit sends an unintended negative message to them instead of acknowledging that they too had a baby of whom they can be proud even if the baby did not live to leave the hospital with them;

  – about the baby's remains. Parents may not know that any tissue removed has to be collected and buried or signed permission given to the hospital to do so;

  – about post-mortems: don't 'force' a post-mortem leaflet on parents.

- **Aftercare**

  Mothers who are physically and emotionally exhausted would welcome on-going support as 'not everyone has friends or a supportive partner to talk to'.

  – Before discharging, talk with both bereaved parents (if possible) and ensure they know where to access help and support should they need it – such as group or one-to-one counselling. Don't take it for granted that people are aware of services.

– An information pack with 'education' about coping and what to what to expect

– emotionally, mentally and physically would be helpful.

– If help is sought through group or one-to-one counselling, let people talk if they want to talk; if they don't want to talk, don't make them talk.

– The GP surgery could check in with a follow-up phone call; offer sympathy for the loss of the baby and ask, 'Do you need anything? Would you like to come in and talk to one of the doctors?'

– A visit from the district midwife – if that service is available to you in your catchment area – would be useful to ensure all is well.

– Hospitals could set up regional monthly Sands meetings for bereaved parents, or meetings with whatever other bereavement support organisations are attached to the particular maternity hospitals Make people aware of the meetings as it would give parents an option.

AWARENESS FOR OTHER PARENTS

- **'A mother's instincts are always right'**
  'You know best, you are the mother, you know your body, you know your baby.'

- **If you have any doubts or concerns** – go and get help; ask the doctor/midwife, keep persisting, ask questions again and again.

- **Get the test** for strep B; get the information if you have any concerns.

- **Be informed:**
  Raise your own awareness: consult the charities via the internet – e.g. gbsaware.co.uk and Count the Kicks. Listen to informative programmes on the radio that focus on stillbirth and miscarriage – a useful form of 'anonymous help'.

  Make yourself aware of everything that is out there to help you before and after.

- **Talk about your baby**
  'Nothing is ever solved by not talking, by not saying anything'; 'You will know in your heart your own way of saying it … I lost a baby at x number of weeks'.

- **Ongoing support of family and friends is very helpful**
  'It was important to have friends and family around … the support we got was incredible and still to this day people talk …'

- **Take mementos of your baby … to have a visual memory**
  'I regret not taking a copy of the baby's scan'; 'I'm sorry I didn't take photos … they offered photographs but I was sort of undecided then … [it would be nice to] have something to look back on but she will always be in my heart'.

- **'Regret not taking our baby home'**
  'I was a little bit worried that the house would become full of memories of … [but] a little bit of me [was] thinking we should probably have taken him home'.

- **Remembering**
  'There are places you can enter your baby's name and have a wee virtual memorial – maybe plant a tree, things that you could do at different stages.'

- **Learn from the past experience**
'If, on reflection, medical care should have been different during the pregnancy, make sure it is different in the future.'

AWARENESS FOR THE GENERAL PUBLIC

- **Permission to grieve**
Understand the huge loss suffered by parents and that every loss has to be grieved. Open up the conversation around miscarriage ... 'it's a painful experience and you want people to "meet" that pain'.

- **Say the baby's name ...** when speaking of him or her.

- **'At least you got to see him'**
'People say to me, "Sure at least you got to see him" – but it doesn't make it any less painful. He was lying there and we had to put him into a coffin.'

- **'You're still young ...'**
'The worst one has got to be "you are both still young, you can still have another baby". If I ever said that to anyone in the past ... make sure I never ever say that again.'

'When people say "sure you are still young, you can have another baby", my first thought is *I don't want another baby ... I want Zach*.'

- **'It's early days; you're lucky you were only 10 weeks'**
People need to know that this message can impinge on the grieving process.

- **'If it was your mother or father who died, people would** commiserate and say, "I'm sorry" ... but if it's a wee baby, people say, "There's your woman her wee baby died" ... I know because I heard people saying it.'

- **'He's not a piece of matter'.**

  'Some people would refer to him as a butterfly baby. It's the process of how the caterpillar becomes a butterfly and can fly away … sometimes those comparisons can niggle at me a little bit'.

- **Sympathy cards**

  The intention is recognised as good but sometimes the message in a card can be 'cold' and have little meaning for parents bereaved of a baby. How could you not stand at a baby's grave and weep?

- **A 'heavenly' perspective helps**

  Belief in an afterlife is soothing. Belief that when a baby dies he or she goes straight to heaven. A book called *Safe in the Arms of God* by American author John MacArthur can be helpful to read.

- **'There is an afterlife'**

  'I do believe that there is an afterlife and that God has plans … my faith has helped me because I do believe that when I die I will be re-united with my children. And that is when I'll find out what God's plan was.'

- **Seek help. Bereavement support is available through Sands, Féileacáin and Cruse Bereavement Care and through other counselling and support organisations**

  – 'Féileacáin have been amazing.'

  – 'Sands parents talk of an acknowledgement of a life.'

  – 'Cruse was my saviour.'

TO RELIGIOUS ORGANISATIONS

- **'Limbo babies'**
  'I can remember a parish priest and when he died he was actually buried with limbo babies because he said he buried so many of them in life, not able to give them a mass. He carried the guilt about that throughout his life. I know now what he meant.'

- **Can the rule be changed to allow a mass for a baby that is lost through miscarriage?**
  'I would have [wanted a mass] but I was told that you don't have that for a miscarried baby. I don't know why and I still don't know 'til this day.'

The information above provides some perspectives on what people valued most in their interactions with healthcare systems as well as what they found difficult. It is hoped that these reflections will provide readers with additional insight into the needs of those who suffer loss.

GLOSSARY

A1C Test
This is a simple blood test that measures a person's average blood sugar levels over a specified period of time.

Acupressure
A form of therapy in which manual pressure is used to stimulate specific points on the body to relieve tension and pain.

Amniotic fluid
The liquid that surrounds the unborn baby during pregnancy.

Ancestors
Family/families of origin from which we have descended.

Antiphospholipid syndrome (APS)
Sometimes known as Hughes syndrome, APS is a disorder of the immune system that causes an increased risk of blood clots. Pregnant women with APS have an increased risk of miscarriage.

Anxiety
Characterised by feeling ill at ease, worried, nervous, tense – often with physical changes, palpitations, breathlessness, increased blood pressure. Having a sense of impending danger, panic or doom.

Arthrogryposis
A term to describe a variety of conditions such as joint stiffness.

Aspirin (and pregnancy)
Low-dose aspirin has been used during pregnancy to reduce the risk of pre-eclampsia in high risk women.

Baptism
The Christian religious ceremony of sprinkling holy water on the forehead and naming a child.

Baptism of the will
If it is the will or desire that a baby is baptised, the baby is considered to be baptised through the will of the parent/s.

Biological clock
The relationship between age and female fertility.

Burial rituals
Different religions and cultures have various ways of honouring their dead depending on their teaching and beliefs. Rituals may include a wake, funeral and cremation.

Catholic tradition
Catholicism revolves around seven sacraments – Baptism, Reconciliation, Eucharist, Confirmation, Marriage, Holy Orders (priesthood), and the Sacrament of the Sick (last rites)

Cervical erosion
Concerns a condition where cells that are found inside the cervical canal are present on the outside surface of the cervix (neck of the womb) cells.

Chicago bloods
Examines if the woman's immune system is attacking the embryos and causing miscarriages.

Chlamydia
A bacterial infection that is sexually transmitted.

Clexane and heparin
Anticoagulants that help prevent blood clots, keep the blood thin.

Clomid
Clomid is one of many fertility drugs on the market. It is administered in certain cases to treat fertility, and issues with ovulation.

Complication
During pregnancy, complications or difficulties may occur due to the health of the mother or the health of the baby.

Conception
Relates to when a child is conceived.

Consultant
In medical terms, a consultant provides expert advice on health and well-being. Usually the most senior grade of hospital doctor and responsible for leading a team.

Cramp
During pregnancy, cramps are said to be common but if they continue they need to be checked by a medical person to ensure that they are not a sign of something more serious.

Cremation
A funeral or post-funeral ritual that some may choose. It is a method of burning the remains and burying the ashes instead of burying the intact dead body.

Depression
A common and serious medical illness that negatively affects how you feel, the way you think and how you act. Among the many traumatic life events that can trigger depression is the loss of a baby.

Dextrocardia
From the Latin word *dexter*, meaning 'right', and Greek *kardia*, meaning 'heart'. It refers to a rare congenital condition in which the apex of the heart is located on the right side of the body.

Diagnosis
The identification of an illness when the symptoms are examined.

Dissociation
The mental process of disconnecting from one's self and the world around you.

Doppler
In pregnancy a doppler is an instrument that is used to carry out a non-invasive imaging test to indicate the baby's blood circulation, uterus and placenta.

DNA and karyotype tests
Genetic tests that identify certain conditions in a baby. A karyotype test looks at the size, shape and number of chromosomes – i.e. parts of cells that contain genes.

Duphaston
A medication used to treat disorders related to the female reproductive cycle.

Ectopic pregnancy
The fertilised egg implants itself outside of the womb, in one of the fallopian tubes that connect the ovaries to the womb.

Embodiment
Concerns the relationship or interaction of our body, our thoughts and our actions.

Emotional support
Providing love, support, reassurance, acceptance and encouragement.

Endrometrial biopsy
In an endometrial biopsy a small piece of tissue from the lining of the uterus (the endometrium) is removed and examined under a microscope.

Estrofem
A hormone replacement therapy that contain an active form of the female hormone, oestrogen.

Fasting insulin
This type of test measures the insulin levels in your blood after at least eight hours of fasting. Insulin is a hormone that regulates how the body absorbs glucose from what we eat.

Flower remedies
Watered-down extracts from the flowers of wild plants – an alternative or complementary treatment used for a variety of conditions including emotional problems and pain.

Foetal akinesia deformation sequence (FADS)
A condition where there is decreased foetal movement.

Foetal assessment unit (FAU)
Offers an assessment to those who need it outside of routine antenatal appointments.

Foetus
In humans, an unborn baby that develops and grows inside the uterus (womb). The fetal period begins 8 weeks after fertilisation of an egg by a sperm and ends at the time of birth.

Fretfulness
A state of being extremely irritable or anxious provoked by worry, irritation or discomfort.

Full-term
The completion of a normal length of pregnancy.

Gabor Maté
A Hungarian-Canadian doctor with a special interest in childhood development and trauma. He believes that addictions originate in trauma and emotional loss.

Gene mutations
Changed or damaged genes. Tests of certain mutations can often determine if the risk of miscarriage is higher.

Gestation
Foetal development period from the time of conception until birth.

Ghost twin
Syndrome where more than one embryo appears to be developing in the womb. At a later stage in the pregnancy the second foetus can no longer be detected.

Hallucinating
Sensations that appear to be real but are created within the mind.

Helplessness
A sense that the person does not have the strength or ability to control a situation.

Homocysteine
A type of amino acid, a chemical that your body uses to make proteins. High levels can cause complications in pregnancy.

Hopelessness
A feeling or state of despair: powerlessness, desperateness.

Insemination
A procedure for treating infertility: sperm are placed directly into the uterus around the time the ovary releases one or more eggs to be fertilised.

In vitro fertilisation (IVF)
A procedure in which eggs are extracted from a woman's ovary and combined with sperm outside the body to form embryos. The embryo is then transferred to the uterus.

Low self-esteem
Defined by lack of confidence, feeling incompetent or inadequate; afraid of making mistakes or letting other people down.

Metaphorical
Something is metaphorical when it stands for or symbolises another thing like a feeling or emotion.

Midwife
A person who is trained to assist women in childbirth.

Miscarriage
Spontaneous or unplanned expulsion of a foetus from the womb before it is able to survive independently.

Mycoplasma and ureaplasma
Tests to check for bacteria in the body that might impact on its ability to conceive.

ORECNI
Office for Research Ethics Committees Northern Ireland

PAI-1
Stands for plasminogen activator inhibitor; an increased PAI-1 is associated with an increased risk for infertility and a worse pregnancy outcome.

Polycystic ovary syndrome (PCOS)
Means that the ovaries have many tiny benign cysts. It due to a combination of genetic and environmental factors. Women with PCOS may also have high testosterone or a lack of ovulation (irregular or no period).

Progesterone
A type of hormone made by the body that plays a role in the menstrual cycle and pregnancy.

Psychological impact
The effect on a person's mental and physical well-being caused by multiple factors including loss and grief, living with chronic or life-limiting medical conditions, relationship problems, accident, injury, man-made or natural disasters.

Psychology
The scientific study of the human mind and behaviour.

Pulsing
A type of therapy to improve health and well-being that may include release of deep physical tension. It is promoted as a gentle and nurturing approach that attempts to increase body awareness and sensitivity.

Rebozo technique
Involves using a scarf or other strong materials to gently rock the woman's body in the hope of bringing relief to the muscles and ligaments around the abdominal and pelvic region.

Reflexology
Massage used to relieve tension and treat illness. The treatment targets reflex points on the feet, hands and head that are linked to every part of the body.

Reiki
Based on the belief that vital energies flows through your body. The Reiki healer will place their hands just above your body to help guide the energies in a way that promotes balance and healing.

Robertsonian balanced translocation
A condition in which there is not enough genetic material for the foetus to continue through pregnancy.

Same-sex relationship
A romantic or sexual relationship between people of the same sex.

Semen analysis
Checks the quality and quantity of the sperm.

Socially constructed
People know and understand life through social interaction and are influenced by socially constructed dominant discourses and societal consensus.

Somatic experiencing (SE)
A body–mind therapeutic approach in the treatment of trauma developed by American psychologist Peter Levine.

Spotting
Refers to very light bleeding that may be experienced at any point in pregnancy.

Stillbirth
When a baby is born dead after twenty-four completed weeks of pregnancy.

Stitch
An intervention to prevent miscarriage, also termed cervical cerclage or cervical stitch.

Strep B infection
A type of bacteria called streptococcal bacteria. If it affects pregnant women it can spread to the unborn baby. As soon as labour begins, antibiotics need to be put into a vein to reduce the risk of the baby getting ill.

Surrogacy
When a woman carries and gives birth to a baby for another person or a couple.

Thyroid function
Measures the levels of thyroid-stimulating hormone (TSH). The thyroid is located in the neck and it produces hormones that regulate growth and development.

Trauma
The response to a deeply distressing or disturbing event that may overwhelm an individual's ability to cope.

Trisomy 18, Edwards syndrome
A chromosomal disorder due to the presence of an extra

chromosome 18. Babies with Trisomy 18 may miscarry or live for only a short time after birth.

Turners syndrome
A genetic condition that affects only females when one of the X chromosomes (sex chromosomes) is missing or partially missing.

Ultrasound scan
During pregnancy, an ultrasound scan is a procedure used to monitor an unborn baby. It uses high-frequency sound waves to create an image of part of the inside of the body.

Umbilical cord
Sometimes referred to as the birth cord, connects the developing embryo with the placenta.

Utrogestan
A medication for women who need extra progesterone while undergoing fertility treatment.

UUREC
Ulster University Research Ethics Committee

Vitamin D, B12 and folate
Vitamin D helps build and maintain healthy bones; B12 helps to keep blood and nerve cells healthy; and folate is important in red blood cell formation and for healthy cell growth and function.

OTHER RESOURCES

It is useful to have knowledge of resources that might be helpful to reach out to in times of need. Those listed below are not intended as recommendations to the readers, but instead comprise some of the services and supports that are currently available throughout the island of Ireland and elsewhere. Additional information on relevant international or regional services may be obtained through their websites. In any situation of concern, readers are advised to seek professional support from their local general practitioner or health authority.

Aisling Centre Enniskillen: **www.theaislingcentre.com**
(Counselling, psychotherapy and well-being service)

A Little Lifetime Foundation: **https://alittlelifetime.ie**
(Provides information and support)

American Psychological Association: **www.apa.org**
(Professional association for psychologists in the United States)

Anam Cara: **https://anamcara.ie**
(Supports parents after a bereavement)

Aware: **www.aware.ie**
(Information and support on fear, anxiety, and depression)

Bereavement Teams – Pregnancy & Infant Loss Ireland: **https://pregnancyandinfantloss.ie/bereavement-teams**
(Bereavement support teams based in maternity hospitals throughout Ireland)

British Psychological Society: **www.bps.org.uk**
(A representative body for psychologists in the United Kingdom)

Canadian Psychological Association: **www.cpa.ca**
(The primary organisation representing psychologists throughout Canada)

Cruse Bereavement Care: **https://www.cruse.org.uk**
(Provides bereavement support to adults and children)

Derry Well Women: **http://www.derrywellwoman.org**
(Offers health and social care services to women of all ages)

Ectopic Pregnancy Ireland: **www.ectopicireland.ie**
(Awareness, information and support)

European Federation of Psychologists' Associations: **www.efpa.eu**
(Umbrella organisation for European psychological associations)

Family Therapy Association of Ireland: **www. familytherapyireland.com**
(Information on therapy for individuals, couples, and families)
Féileacáin: **https://feileacain.ie**
(Provides support to anyone affected by the death of a baby during or after pregnancy)

Irish Association for Counselling and Psychotherapy: **www.iacp.ie**
(Professional association for counsellors and psychotherapists)

Irish Council for Psychotherapy (ICP): **www. psychotherapycouncil.ie**
(The national umbrella body for psychotherapy in Ireland, ICP also acts as a link between those who are looking for psychotherapy services and those who provide them)

Irish Hospice Foundation: **http://hospicefoundation.ie**
(Bereavement support line in partnership with the HSE)

Kicks Count: **http://www.kickscount.org.uk**
(UK's leading foetal movement awareness campaign)

Life After Loss: **http://www.lifeafterloss.org.uk**
(Facebook group; support and information)

Mariposa Trust: **https://www.mariposatrust.org**
(Baby loss information and support)

Mental Health Ireland: **www.mentalhealthireland.ie**
(Advocacy and support for mental health)

MindYourSelf Series: **mindyourselfbooks.ie**
(Safe, researched, peer-reviewed self-care, health and well-being book series)

Miscarriage Association of Ireland: **https://miscarriage.ie**
(Helpline and support meetings)

Miscarriage Association UK: **www.miscarriageassociation.org.uk**
(Helpline, online support, support groups, information)

Pregnancy Loss Message Board: **https://rollercoaster.ie/community/pregnancy-loss**
(Discussion forum on topics related to pregnancy loss)

Pregnancy & Infant Loss Ireland: **https://pregnancyandinfantloss.ie**
(Directory of support services and knowledge for bereaved parents and health professionals)

Psychological Society of Ireland: **www.psychologicalsociety.ie**
(Professional body for psychologists and psychology in the Republic of Ireland)

Rainbows Ireland: **www.rainbowsireland.ie**
(Supporting parents to support bereaved children)

Samaritans, Ireland: **https://www.samaritans.org/ireland/
samaritans-ireland**
(Emotional support 24 hours per day – phone helpline, email,
face-to-face support and outreach in communities, schools)

Samaritans, UK: **https://www.samaritans.org**
(Listening and support for people and communities in times of
need)

Sands Bereavement Care: **https://www.sands.org.uk**
(Bereavement support services through freephone helpline, mobile
app, online community and resources)

SiMBA: **https://www.simbacharity.org.uk**
(Range of supports and services including birth acknowledgement
certificates)

OTHER READING

Stillbirth and Miscarriage, a Life-changing Loss: 'Say my baby's name' is based on the lived experience of the mums and dads who courageously shared their stories of loss. The book also incorporates research, wisdom and insights from other sources. There is a wealth of relevant material in the form of books, papers and poetry, by Irish writers and further afield. The aim of the list below is to provide a range of options for those who wish to continue reading about the important topic of stillbirth and miscarriage.

Abboud, L.N. and Liamputtong, P., 'Pregnancy Loss: What it means to women who miscarry and their partners', *Social Work in Health Care*, vol. 36, no. 3, 2003, pp. 37–62

Bateman, L., Jones, C. and Jomeen, J., 'A Narrative Synthesis of Women's Out-of-Body Experiences During Childbirth', *Journal of Midwifery & Women's Health*, vol. 62, 2017, pp. 442–51, https://doi.org/10.1111/jmwh.12655

Brier, N., 'Grief Following Miscarriage: A comprehensive review of the literature', *Journal of Women's Health*, vol. 17, no. 3, 2008, pp. 451–64

Burden, C., Bradley, S., Storey, C., Ellis, A., Heazell, A.E.P., Downe, S., Cacciatore, J. and Siassakos, D., 'From Grief, Guilt Pain and Stigma to Hope and Pride: A systematic review and meta-analysis of mixed-method research of the psychosocial impact of stillbirth', *BMC Pregnancy and Childbirth*, vol. 16, no. 9, 2016, https://doi.org/10.1186/s12884-016-0800-8

Campbell-Jackson, L. and Horsch, A., 'The Psychological Impact of Stillbirth on Women: A systematic review', *Illness, Crisis & Loss*, vol. 22, no. 3, 2014, pp. 237–56

Campbell-Jackson, L., Bezance, J. and Horsch, A., '"A Renewed Sense of Purpose": Mothers' and fathers' experience of having a child following a recent stillbirth', *BMC Pregnancy and Childbirth,* vol. 14, 2014, http://doi.org/10.1186/s12884-014-0423-x

Cantrell, J., *Carried Within Me: Echoes of infant loss from bereaved parents* (Pittsburgh, PA: Lighthouse Point Press, 2019)

Cecil, R., 'Memories of Pregnancy Loss: Recollections of elderly women in Northern Ireland', in R. Cecil (ed.), *The Anthropology of Pregnancy Loss: Comparative studies in miscarriage, stillbirth and neonatal death* (Oxford: Berg, 1996)

Colgan, K., *If It Happens To You: Miscarriage and stillbirth – a human insight* (Dublin: A&A Farmar, 1994)

Corry, D.A., Tracey, A.P. and Lewis, C.A., 'Spirituality and Creativity in Coping, Their Association and Transformative Effect: A qualitative enquiry', *Religions*, vol. 6, no. 2, 2015, pp. 499–526, https://doi.org/10.3390/rel6020499

Cullen, S., Coughlan, B., Casey, B., Power, S. and Brosnan, M., 'Exploring Parents' Experiences of Care in an Irish Hospital Following a Second-Trimester Miscarriage', *British Journal of Midwifery*, vol. 25, vol. 2, 2018, pp. 110–15

Draper, J., '"It Was a Real Good Show": The ultrasound scan, fathers and the power of visual knowledge', *Sociology of Health and Illness*, vol. 24, no. 6, 2002, pp. 771–95

Due, C., Chiarolli, S. and Riggs, D.W. 'The Impact of Pregnancy Loss on Men's Health and Well-Being: A systematic review', *BMC Pregnancy and Childbirth,* vol. 17, 2017

Gourney, K. and Ashcroft, B., *Hope and Healing after Stillbirth and New Baby Loss* (London: John Murray Press, 2019)

Greenhalgh, T., 'Narrative-Based Medicine in an Evidence-Based World', *British Medical Journal*, vol. 318, no. 7179, 1999, pp. 323–5

Heaney, S., 'Elegy for a Still-Born Child', in Siobhan Parkinson (ed.), *A Part of Ourselves: Laments for lives that ended too soon* (Dublin: A&A Farmar, 1997), p. 99.

Johnston, M., 'Road's End', in *The Whetstone* (Kilcar, Co. Donegal: Summer Palace Press, 2019), p. 57

Kahn, M., *Whatever Arises, Love That: A love revolution that begins with you* (Louisville, CO: Sounds True, 2016)

Keenan, B. 'Trauma Is a Fact of Life But It Doesn't Have To Be a Life Sentence', https://iahip.org/page-1075484 (Irish Association of Integrative and Humanistic Psychotherapy)

Kubler-Ross, E., *On Death and Dying* (New York: Macmillan, 1969)

Lee C. and Rowlands, I.J., 'When Mixed Methods Produce Mixed Results: Integrating disparate findings about miscarriage and women's wellbeing', *British Journal of Health Psychology,* vol. 20, 2015, pp. 36–44

Levine, P.A. with Frederick, A., *Waking the Tiger: Healing trauma* (Berkeley, CA: North Atlantic Books, 1997)

MacArthur, John, *Safe in the Arms of God* (Nashville: Thomas Nelson, 2003)

Maté, G., *When the Body Says No: Exploring the stress–disease connection* (New Jersey: John Wiley & Sons Inc., 2003)

McCreight, B.S., 'Perinatal Loss: A qualitative study in Northern Ireland', *OMEGA*, vol. 57, no. 1, 2008, pp. 1–19

McCreight, B.S., 'Narratives of Pregnancy Loss: The role of self-help groups in supporting parents', *Medical Sociology Online*, vol. 2, no. 1, 2007, pp. 3–16

McCreight, B.S., 'Perinatal Grief and Emotional Labour: A study of nurses' experiences in gynae wards', *International Journal of Nursing Studies*, vol. 42, no. 4, 2005, pp. 439–48

McCreight, B.S., 'A Grief Ignored: Narratives of pregnancy loss from a male perspective', *Sociology of Health & Illness*, vol. 26, no. 3, 2004, pp. 273–383

McGovern, M. and Tracey, A., 'A Comparative Examination of Schools' Responses to Bereavement and the Associated Needs of the School Community in Galway, West of Ireland and Derry, Northern Ireland', *Pastoral Care in Education*, vol. 28, no. 3, 2010, pp. 235–52

McGreal, D., Evans, B.J. and Burrows, G.D., 'Gender Differences in Coping Following Loss of a Child Through Miscarriage or Stillbirth: A pilot study', *Stress Medicine*, vol. 13, no. 3, 1997, pp. 139–207

Meaney, M.A., Everard, C.M., Gallagher, S. and O'Donoghue, K., 'Parents' Concerns about Future Pregnancy after Stillbirth: A qualitative study', *Health Expectations*, vol. 20, no. 4, 2017, pp. 555–62

Mulvihill, A. and Walsh, T., 'Pregnancy Loss in Rural Ireland: An experience of disenfranchised grief', *British Journal of Social Work*, vol. 44, 2014, pp. 2290–2306

Murphy, S., Shevlin, M. and Elklit, A., 'Psychological Consequences of Pregnancy Loss and Infant Death in a Sample of Bereaved Parents', *Journal of Loss and Trauma*, vol. 19, no. 1, 2014, pp. 56–69, http://dx.doi.org/10.1080/15325024.2012.735531

O'Connell, M.A., Leahy-Warren, P., Kenny, L.C., O'Neill, S.M. and Khashan, A.S., 'The Prevalence and Risk Factors of Fear of Childbirth Among Pregnant Women: A cross-sectional study in Ireland', AOGS [Acta Obstetricia et Gynecologica Scandinavica], vol. 98, no. 8, 2019, pp. 1014–23, https://doi.org/10.1111/aogs.13599

Pais, M. and Pai, M.V., 'Stress Among Pregnant Women: A systematic review', *Journal of Clinical and Diagnostic Research*, vol. 12, no. 5, 2018, pp. 1–4

Parkinson, S., *All Shining in the Spring: The story of a baby who died* (Dublin: Little Island Books, 2021)

Peters, M.D.J., Lisy, K., Riitano, D., Jordan, Z. and Aromataris, E., 'Caring for Families Experiencing Stillbirth: Evidence-based guidance for maternity care providers', *Women and Birth*, vol. 28, no. 4, 2015, pp. 272–8

Rothert, D., *At a Loss: Finding your way after miscarriage, stillbirth or infant death* (New York: Open Air Books, 2019)

Tracey, A., *Surviving the Early Loss of a Mother: Daughters speak* (Dublin: Veritas, 2008)

Tracey, A. and Holland, J., 'A Comparative Study of the Child Bereavement and Loss Responses and Needs of Schools in Hull, Yorkshire and Derry/Londonderry, Northern Ireland', *Pastoral Care in Education*, vol. 26, no. 4, 2008, pp. 253–66

van der Kolk, B., *The Body Keeps the Score: Brain, mind and body in the healing of trauma* (New York: Viking Press, 2014)

Williams, H.M., Jones L.L., Coomarasamy, A. and Topping, A.E., 'Men Living Through Multiple Miscarriages: Protocol for a qualitative exploration of experiences and support requirements', *British Medical Journal* (2020), https://bmjopen.bmj.com/content/10/5/e035967

Williams, H.M., Jones L.L., Coomarasamy, A. and Topping, A.E., 'Men and Miscarriage: A systematic review and thematic synthesis', *Qualitative Health Research*, vol. 30, no. 1, 2019, pp. 133–45

Worden, W., *Grief Counselling and Grief Therapy: A handbook for the mental health practitioner*, 2nd edn (London: Routledge, 1996)

Wright, E., *Ask Me His Name: Learning to live and laugh again after the loss of my baby* (Sweden: Lagom, 2019)

INDEX